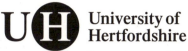
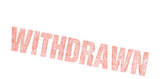

The International Library of Group Analysis
Edited by Malcolm Pines, Institute of Group Analysis, London

The aim of this series is to represent innovative work in group psychotherapy, particularly but not exclusively group analysis. Group analysis, taught and practised widely in Europe, has developed from the work of S.H. Foulkes.

other titles in the series

Circular Reflections
Selected Papers on Group Analysis and Psychoanalysis
Malcolm Pines
ISBN 1 85302 492 9 pb
ISBN 1 85302 493 7 hb
International Library of Group Analysis 1

Foundations and Applications of Group Psychotherapy
A Sphere of Influence
Mark F. Ettin
ISBN 1 85302 795 2
International Library of Group Analysis 10

Taking the Group Seriously
Towards a Post-Foulkesian Group Analytic Theory
Farhad Dalal
ISBN 1 85302 642 5
International Library of Group Analysis 5

of related interest

Bion, Rickman and Foulkes and the Northfield Experiments
Advancing to a Different Front
Tom Harrison
ISBN 1 85302 837 1
Therapeutic Communities 5

Introduction to Therapeutic Communites
David Kennard
ISBN 1 85302 603 4
Therapeutic Communities 1

Dialogue in the Analytic Setting
Selected Papers of Louis Zinkin on Jung and on Group Analysis
Edited by Hindle Zinkin, Rosemary Gordon and Jane Haynes
ISBN 1 85302 610 7

The Challenge for Psychoanalysis and Psychotherapy
Solutions for the Future
Edited by Stefan de Schill and Serge Lebovici
ISBN 1 85302 477 5

INTERNATIONAL LIBRARY OF GROUP ANALYSIS 12

A Century of Psychiatry, Psychotherapy and Group Analysis

A Search for Integration

Ronald Sandison

Foreword by Malcolm Pines

Jessica Kingsley Publishers
London and Philadelphia

The identity of the photographer who took the pictures on pp.48–49 in not known. If anyone knows of his or her whereabouts, we would be grateful if they could come forward so that his or her permission for their use can be sought.

All reasonable effort has been made to contact Norman MacKenzie who took the photograph on p.50 to obtain his permission for its use. It is included here as it was in his own publication *Dreams and Dreaming* (1965) published by Aldus Books in London.

The photograph on p.110 entitled *The Great Nebula (M31) in Andromeda* is reprinted here as it appeared as Plate IV opposite p.30 in *The Universe Around Us* (1929) by James Jeans, published by Cambridge University Press, with the kind permission of the Yerkes Laboratory at the University of Chicago.

First published in the United Kingdom in 2001 by
Jessica Kingsley Publishers Ltd
116 Pentonville Road
London N1 9JB, England
and
325 Chestnut Street
Philadelphia, PA 19106, USA

www.jkp.com

Copyright © 2001 Ronald Sandison

Library of Congress Cataloging in Publication Data
A CIP catalog record for this book is available from the Library of Congress

British Library Cataloguing in Publication Data
A CIP catalogue record for this book is available from the British Library

ISBN 1 85302 869 X

Printed and Bound in Great Britain by
Athenaeum Press, Gateshead, Tyne and Wear

Contents

Preface

My career in psychiatry began in 1946, after I left the Royal Air Force. Fifty years later, in 1996, I began to think about writing a book concerning some of the experiences of my professional life. Psychotherapy has always been uppermost in my mind as the prime agent for healing in my engagement with my patients. Through the years I had written a fair number of papers on whatever aspect of the subject was gripping me at the time. At one stage in my musing I had an idea of putting them together as a collected volume. Such collections seldom give a clear idea of the growth and development of either the author or the maturity of his work, so I abandoned the notion.

I decided that what I needed was a context for the growth of my ideas about human interaction and the human psyche. Some of my colleagues have done this through using 'places and people' as their context. The series 'In Conversation with...' in the *Bulletin of the British Journal of Psychiatry* is an example. However, one learns little or nothing about the psychiatrist as a human being. Traditionally, doctors, being shamans and therefore apart from other men, were not allowed to have private lives, private thoughts or human weaknesses. This tradition lives on, fostered by the expectations of patients and acted out by doctors themselves. For example, doctors are never supposed to be ill, to have family lives, or to need rest or recreation. They should be always there, and as alert and resourceful at two in the morning as at all other times.

Psychotherapy is based on the relationship between two people. The patient is not expected to know anything about the analyst as a person, while revealing all him or herself. As I hope to show, the personality of the therapist is coded in his consulting room and its contents, and in his presence and being with the patient. The journals and textbooks are full of descriptive and analytical accounts of the work of psychotherapists. When reading them I long to know more about the person who wrote the words. The rules which govern self-disclosure in the consulting room seem to hold good for the printed word as well.

After several trials I decided that the only way of making sense of what I had done in the various fields in which I have worked over the years was to provide it with a context. It had to be more than 'places and people'. So what follows in this book is autobiographical whenever appropriate. If I appear to get carried away into areas remote from the psychotherapeutic text at times, I can only reply that what is intensely important to me necessarily becomes part of my psychotherapeutic self. In the course of a varied, and to me interesting, career, I have been seeking a unifying principle. I find that in my own history.

The title of this book is not intended to convey the idea that I have written a history of psychotherapy through the 20th century. I have made the rather bold assumption that the principles and practice of psychoanalysis and its derivatives is one of the few, if not the only, truly unifying factors in this century of vast social, material and spiritual change and upheaval. I lived through all but 16 years of that century, and its upheavals were reflected in my own life. For me also, my understanding of the unconscious has been my own unifying principle. I hope that the exercise of this has helped a few other people, my patients, in their own journeys.

Jung was not able to reveal any of his own biographical details in print until he wrote *Memories, Dreams, Reflections*, at the age of 83 (Jung 1961). Even so, it was left to his many biographers subsequently to tease out aspects of his life which he did not care to enlarge on. Few analysts have followed Jung's example. While I was thinking about what to write in my preface I chanced on a paper by Joyce McDougall in the *Journal of Analytical Psychology*. There she describes in frank detail her reasons for seeking analysis herself (McDougall 2000). I applaud her courage in taking, what to me appears to be, a considerable risk. On reflection I wonder whether this feeling is not yet another wish on my part to hold on to the image of the doctor or healer as a semi-divine being.

Biographies tend to be long and weighty tomes. I am conscious that in this relatively short account of my life and work I have had to omit so much. Even now that the work is 'finished', memories tug at my sleeve asking plaintively why they were not included. It has been essential to keep important parts of myself as my own, they are not to go on display. I keep them for my own stability, they behave like ballast on a small boat. In any case, they have more meaning to me than to others. That at least is my belief.

My thanks are due to many. In particular to Malcolm Pines whom I have known for well over 30 years. He patiently read my earlier drafts and encouraged me to adopt the autobiographical mode. His encouragement and suggestions have been an invaluable spur, and given me the courage to complete the task. I would like to thank him also, as editor of *Group Analysis*, for permission to reproduce extensive extracts from my sum of papers that have been published there over the years. He has generously written the foreword to this book. My thanks also go to Dr Douglas Haldane, a former consultant at the Ross Clinic, Aberdeen, who kindly read the chapter 'Shetland and Aberdeen', and thus enabled me to avoid some errors. Many friends and colleagues have commented and encouraged me, and thus provided more support than they knew.

Every word of every draft has been patiently listened to by my wife, Beth, whose judgement and criticism I greatly value. Our lives have been curiously intertwined for over 30 years. This book is not all about me, there is a lot of Beth secretly hidden in it also. Finally, I feel it is prudent to remember the muse, which one I will not name, who has been my constant companion in this task during the past two years. As well as being a good friend, she has also been a demanding mistress, but she has not deserted me. I hope she will share my feeling now that she can have a rest for a time, but I do not wish her to desert me.

Foreword

Ronnie Sandison was born in the Shetland Islands, in the far north of Scotland, where his family had lived for hundreds of years. Though in his early childhood his family had moved south, nevertheless he has been at home in sea and air, the elements of his island home. He has sailed, fished, explored the physiology of the air of rapid altitude ascents in Spitfires during the 1939–45 war, knows the false euphoria of oxygen lack. As a psychiatrist using LSD in psychotherapy, he has also known the false euphoria of pharmacotherapy and returned to the slow humane exploration of the psyche, using a psychoanalytic psychotherapy informed by Freud's psychoanalysis, Jung's analytical psychology and finally Foulkes' group analysis.

Ronnie Sandison's autobiography is a valuable documentation of the state of psychiatry in the United Kingdom in the second half of the twentieth century. There can be few such as he who attended lectures by J.A. Hadfield, a now forgotten but then important figure in the formative years of psychoanalysis in London, who was influential in the Tavistock Clinic and first analyst to W.R. Bion. T.P. Rees, a powerful force for progress in mental hospital psychiatry at Warlingham Park, inspired Sandison in his turn to breathe new life into a run-down mental hospital. He toured Europe to explore new approaches, pioneered LSD treatment; he established a new psychiatric service in the Shetlands, fostered psychotherapy in the south-west of England at Southampton, and finally brought his psychodynamic approach to his work in birth control and fertility clinics.

Ronnie Sandison's dreams have been his life-compass, foretelling him of dangers, and showing him opportunities. He is a talented dreamer; I admire, and also envy, the deep understanding he derives from his dream life. He learnt to trust his unconscious in a way that is a model to us and has enabled his patients to trust their own messages from the unconscious. Thereby I understand his being at home with Foulkes' group analysis, for Foulkes also had a deep trust of the emerging wisdom of properly conducted group analysis.

I am privileged to have been asked to write a foreword to this fine, wise, generous book. I have seen its gradual emergence as Ronnie, in his eighties, happily married to Beth, has drawn on his life experience with his excellent memory (much better than mine in my mid-seventies) and looks over his more than half century of experience in psychiatry and psychotherapy. He draws us into seeing the world as he found it, and changed it.

Louis Zinkin, his Jungian analyst, whom he loved and from whom he learnt much, was a friend and colleague of mine at school and later in psychiatry and group analysis. I am glad for this sensitive glimpse of Louis at work.

Ronnie Sandison is glad for his many, varied, colourful life experiences. He has woven them into a rich fabric.

His life journey has found a good harbour.

Malcolm Pines
May 2000

CHAPTER 1

Beginnings

I was born in 1916, not long before the commencement of the Battle of the Somme which raged from July to November and dominated the lives and thoughts of almost every family in the land. I was quite unconscious of these events, despite the fact that three of my uncles were at the front, and most of my other male and some female relatives were at war. I am sure that my mother was unaware of the psychodynamic work for 'shell-shocked' officers being done by William Rivers at Craiglockhart Hospital, or that Sigmund Freud had at least 20 creative years of work to his credit, or that Carl Jung, after the break with Freud, was making his most profound discoveries. My belief is that what entered my consciousness and passed into my unconscious were my mother's joint fears of starvation and Zeppelins. Of these she would talk after the war when I was older, and in those days she soothed my night terrors with stories, among which the Angels of Mons stays in my memory. She was a great believer in angels and especially in a personal guardian angel. After a long life I not only share her belief, I know.

These early events took place in the Shetland Isles, 200 miles north of Aberdeen and halfway to the Faroe Islands. My mother was English, and my father was a Shetlander whose family was descended from a long line known to stretch back to the 15th century, and well documented since 1681. My early years were dominated by a huge weight of ancestral stories from his family which I found alternately oppressive and exciting. My father's image contrasted strongly with that of my mother. My earliest recollections of him are derived almost entirely from the objects around him and his gifts to me. For example, from the age of two his model yacht, made by a local boat-builder, was my constant companion. He communicated with me through these objects, and his books. His world was an inner one, and books were his companions.

The range of subjects on the shelves was wide, but I knew that the authors who really touched him were otherworldly. George MacDonald (1949), Sheridan le Fanu, M.R. James, Edgar Allan Poe and Algernon Blackwood were among them. These authors portrayed a world ranging from indescribable beauty to great horror and demonic possession, but always with a sense of reincarnation or *déjà vu*. They were part of his secret life, revealed to me only in milli-seconds of contact with his mind. For example, when I told him that we were reading *The Princess and the Goblin* at Kindergarten a strange light came into his eyes, and a couple of days later he arrived home with that and its sequel, *The Princess and Curdy*, which he handed to me without a word. These stories of good and evil introduced me to a fundamental subject with which I have spent the rest of my life wrestling.

This mystical insight into my father's inner life, donated in widely separated flashes of insight, did not characterise my everyday dealings with him. My experience of what Jung would call his number 1 personality was the wonder of hearing him read Kipling's *Just So Stories* (1918) and others when I was five years old. He was a good reader and an excellent mimic, and read *The Pickwick Papers* (Dickens 1892) aloud to perfection. I enjoyed these many readings, but I inwardly knew that they did not proceed from the person I longed to know. I needed another role model. I found it, I thought, in my Uncle Jack, but even he did not satisfy some indefinable longing which led me to many years of searching.

There are many different ways of telling the story of my early years, and some of them will be found in this book. I offer here one path. Taking it led to developments that have occupied me for the rest of my life. Uncle Jack was both known and unknown to me. He was born in 1875 and qualified in medicine at Edinburgh about the turn of the century. By that time he had travelled extensively in Europe and the Far East, many photographs of which are still extant. I know little about his life until the First World War began, except that he married and that his wife died in 1905 giving birth to their only child, Ian. In 1919 he married my father's eldest sister and entered our family story. He was a great narrative teller, and I remember him best when I was young when he would stand in front of the fire and tell long engaging tales of travel and adventure. Of course, his stories about his steam cars intrigued me most. But, in those troubled post-war days, he would most often talk about the war. He had been in Gallipoli, and after the evacuation he spent the rest of the war on the Western Front. What stories they were! And among my most treasured possessions are his boxes of medicines and antiseptics, and some of his instruments which went with him and were used there. Most poignant of all is his brass pocket compass, made in France, which must have served him well on many occasions. In poor health after the war he was appointed the first Medical Officer of Health (MOH) in Shetland in 1919, a post which he held for ten years, retiring in 1929 to Tayvallich in Argyll, a place he had known and loved as a boy.

Being MOH of Shetland was not the administrative desk-bound job that it is today. Jack travelled extensively. There are over 100 islands in the Shetland group, and probably 40 of them were inhabited in his day, some by only one crofting family. Whenever a doctor was needed, or there was an epidemic, he was there, and again this generated many stories which made him a doctor-hero in my eyes. He was a great man for experimenting, mostly with food, as he was quite sure that he knew how Britain could feed itself in the event of another world conflict. He was certain that it would come although he did not live to see it. During those years in Shetland he saw a lot of Sir William Watson Cheyne, who had returned to his boyhood home on the island of Fetlar in 1919, where he lived until his death in 1932. Cheyne had been Joseph Lister's assistant in Edinburgh, had gone with him to King's in London, and succeeded as senior surgeon when Lister retired. Watson Cheyne had an interesting connection with our family. His father Andrew had been educated by my great-great-grandfather at Tangwick in Eshaness where he ran a school for 50 years. The childhoods of both Andrew and William are such as to excite the interest of psychotherapists. Andrew was the illegitimate son of the laird's brother, and was brought up in the 'big house', thus having an absent mother and two fathers. He spent his adult life opening up the sandalwood trade in the Pacific Ocean until he was murdered on Koror in 1866. It was only then, aged 13, that William learned who his father was, having been brought up in the minister's family as William Watson. Yet, and perhaps because of this, he had a brilliant career, living out the endless searching for fame which had been denied his father.

Of course I remember Uncle Jack in Shetland. I well remember sitting in a room in the turret of his home which I made my own and gazing out over Fort Charlotte and the harbour of Lerwick. But it is the days and weeks I spent in Tayvallich from the age of nine onwards which are etched deepest in my memory. At home in London I had my telescope and my weather station, but in Tayvallich, Loch Sween was my playground, and the whole of nature came to life in those long summer days. The house was a centre for the many students, mostly of Natural Science, who came each summer and generously included me in some of their expeditions. Several held chairs in later years. But it was in my teenage years, after Jack retired, that he gave me what my father could have given, but never quite seemed able to.

We would set out in the morning, he and I, rowing the dinghy to the furthest reaches of the loch, and spend a long day talking and collecting seaweed and plants. He brought a dimension to our family which I had known only from schoolmasters. He loved the classics with a passion which transcended anything I had known before. Sometimes at home he would read part of a tragedy in the original Greek, and it always brought a tear to my eye. Sometimes he would read Virgil, also in the original, and the great rolling lines of the *Aeneid* took me into the very centre of the heroic age. He wrote a number of plays in his last years, mostly about Bonnie Prince Charlie and the Jacobites. Again the poetry of lines like 'And then sadness and despair came upon me like the mist drifting low over the hills', punctuating the text at intervals, entered deep into my memory. Those plays are lost to me now, but their memory remains fresh. In our private moments I knew that he, like my father, had an otherworldly dimension to his mind. My father resonated with it, but Jack lived it. During the war, he told me, one of the nursing sisters on his unit had fallen into a sort of depressive decline, and was eventually admitted to hospital. Visiting her there she told him that it was all due to her having accepted a 'bad-luck' ring from one of her patients. Jack said simply 'Give me the ring', which she did. He told me that everything went wrong for him after that, and that it took him months to regain his equilibrium. It was a chilling story. My father read stories like W.W. Jacob's *Monkey's Paw* (1924); Uncle Jack lived them out.

I know that it was Jack who gave me permission to explore the unconscious, and to study medicine. I know also that he never made a single suggestion about what I should do for a career. Sadly, he did not live to see what I made of our time together, as he died in 1935, a year after I started pre-clinical studies. He left me his telescope, his barometer, some of his medical instruments, a collection of ophthalmoscopes, and most wonderful of all, his Leitz microscope and a number of books. Some of the latter reflect our common interests, especially Eder's translation (Undated) of Freud's second edition of *The Interpretation of Dreams*, which may well be the first time Freud's original writing appeared in English. Pettigrew's *Medical Superstitions* (1844) and a book on mediaeval witchcraft, *Demonology* (now lost), reflected his interest in folk stories and mythology, as did Norman Macrae's *Highland Second Sight* (1908) and Northcote Thomas's *Thought Transference: A Critical and Historical Review of the Evidence for Telepathy, 1902–1903* (1905). A curiosity is Sir Arthur Mitchell's *About Dreaming, Laughing and Blushing* (1905), a pre-Freudian attempt by a psychiatrist to account for these uniquely human attributes. Laughing, according to him, is a form of temporary insanity. Perhaps this dour Scottish author did not laugh very much. Laughter was a subject which appealed to Jack, and the only surviving manuscript of his in my possession consists of notes he made for a lecture on 'Laughter'. The joining of the light-hearted to the scholarly describes the man I knew. In the lecture he moves from a study of tickling and of the effects of laughing gas (nitrous oxide), as promoters of laughter, through examples of 'Irish Bulls' to an invocation of the works of philosophers down the ages, including Aristotle, Hobbes, Bain, Kant and Schopenhauer. These notes are very tantalising, as they are laced with headings for stories. How I wish I could have heard the lecture! Differing from Mitchell, he thought of laughter as a form of play begun in childhood. But it was the microscope which I valued most and used extensively during my student years. It was a beautiful instrument, rather antiquated by today's standards, but what an astonishing world was revealed to me through its lenses.

When I was about 16, Jack and I spent one of our long days in the boat. On that day he talked about girls and nothing else. He talked with a kind of passion which I found quite alarming at times. It was an experience which was deeply disturbing to my life which had been spent hitherto in an almost exclusively male world, apart from the women at home, my mother, grandmother and servants. This was not a 'father to son' talk about the facts of life; it was a deeply passionate discourse on the need for the feminine in a man's life. Over and over again he would say, 'Girls, girls, girls, you must have them, always, always, always.' It was like an invitation to enter one of Hermann Hesse's fantasies of women. In a rare revelation about his own early life he said something like, 'You must have girls, girls, girls; I never kissed a girl until I was 15, and she was my cousin.' At 16 I hadn't kissed a girl, and his urging, in the context of nearly 70 years ago, was timely. I do not think that I immediately took his advice literally, but something about that day, melded with all my other experience of him, set me on the way to find the feminine in myself. To achieve this I had to know much more about the inner world of women themselves.

In 1945, ten years after Uncle Jack died, I was about to leave the Royal Air Force, where I had served as a physiologist for over five years, and in the following year I joined the staff as a trainee psychiatrist at Warlingham Park Hospital, Surrey. My working world had been almost exclusively male until then, and it seemed destined to remain that way, as I was assigned to the male side of the hospital, under the senior medical officer. By tradition the women's side was in the hands of the deputy medical superintendent. Dr William Shepley was a self-taught Freudian analyst, who had a bunch of young women patients who lived in one of the four villas, α-house. He shared this territory with an orthodox Freudian, Dr Joyce Martin, who was less flamboyant than Shepley about her style of analysis. Their counterpart on the male side was Dennis Scott, a Jungian analyst in training, and in analysis with Michael Fordham. There were three other women on the medical staff. In the medical mess I began to hear words like 'anima', 'the self' and 'mandala' as part of the currency of mealtime discussions. I warmed towards the Jungians, and yearned to experience for myself this inner world of women that Uncle Jack had urged me to explore and make part of my life more than ten years earlier.

At that stage of my career the male psyche did not interest me greatly. I duly spent time with my male patients and tried to get to know and understand them, but it was the mystery of women that I had an imperative need to fathom. Fortunately the hospital system was very flexible, and I spent a lot of time in the female insulin room, exploring the fantasies and dreams of the patients before, during and after coma. Once I had established my desire to follow the analytical path,

William Shepley was happy for me to take on any women patients I admitted whom I thought I could help. I hadn't much faith in him as a supervisor, so I went my own way. Dr T.P. Rees, the medical superintendent, a man of great intuition and keen to promote the idiosyncrasies and interests of the junior staff, began to refer patients to me for therapy. Curiously enough, they all turned out to be young women, and I received much sound practical advice under his supervision.

Entering this new world left me with many regrets for what I appeared to be abandoning. My medical training had given me a desire to assemble and sift facts, to reach a diagnosis, to search for the unusual and the obscure, and to match the diagnosis with a treatment plan. My concept of the importance of the doctor himself was not easy to understand as being part of being a 'proper doctor'. My biggest inhibition came from the fact that I was working in an asylum. It is true that it was actually called a mental hospital, but to the local people and to most of the people I met socially, it was where the mad people went, and mad people were aliens. The medical superintendent was the enlightened and charismatic Percy Rees. The formation of his famous 'barrow squads' as one means of giving patients some useful activity did nothing to dispel this image of alienation. The lines of long-stay patients moving about the grounds were reminders that these were the results of failure, as most of them would spend the rest of their lives in the hospital.

One of my early discoveries was that there were, in the minds of the doctors, two kinds of patient: neurotic and psychotic. The policy of admitting as many patients as possible on a voluntary basis and the strong analytical presence among the doctors resulted in there being two hospitals side by side. The neurotics were the 'villa patients' and the newly admitted psychotics and the long-stay patients were in the main building. The villa patients received psychotherapy, those in the wards received their 'treatment' at a distance, as it were. Physical treatments such as electro-convulsive therapy (ECT) and insulin coma therapy were at the height of their popularity, whilst the long-stay patients were still being dosed with chloral hydrate and paraldehyde, known as the 'draught and powder', or with bromide and valerian. There were two wards whose patients were nearly all epileptic and being treated with the recently developed drug epanutin. This controlled their fits and perhaps prevented further mental deterioration, but did nothing for their personalities. Rees was acutely aware of the need to improve the lot of the long-stay patients and much of his energy was directed there. The barrow parties had been introduced before the war, and during my time between 1946 and 1951 the medical staff was increased by the appointment of several very able doctors whose work transformed these wards. Among these were Arthur Zanker and Sydney Mitchell. Zanker was a refugee from Austria who had trained under Alfred Adler, and had a special interest in child psychiatry. Both he and

Mitchell were musicians, and Arthur had been a member of the Vienna Symphony Orchestra in happier times.

They discovered much musical talent among the long-stay patients and their orchestra gave lunch-hour concerts. They had gramophone recitals, and therapy groups were formed around music themes. Their paper was published in October 1948. After giving a scholarly survey of the use of music in emotionally disturbed people from the time of Pythagoras onwards, they concluded that traditional and folk music were the most effective means of promoting harmony and integration of the group as a whole. Being classical musicians themselves, I detect some disappointment from their finding that romantic and classical music did not lead to the same results. There is a continuing literature on the use of music in therapy, and a more recent paper by Andrew Powell (1981) is a good example of ways of understanding group dynamics through musical metaphor.

For me, my abiding memory of Mitchell and Zanker's work is that of the orchestra. The pianist was accomplished and a fairly recent admission to the hospital. The violinist, however, was a lady nearing 80 years of age who had been in the hospital for many years. She had, in the far distant past, been a concert violinist, but had never played since. Miraculously, her violin was found, and she regained much of her early skill. Zanker might play his cello, and the bulk of the orchestra was made up of cymbals and other percussion instruments, mouth organs, nightingales and drums. Mitchell himself scored various pieces to suit this rather strange collection of instruments, and conducted the group. It was a most moving affair, and those concerts remain in my memory as a memorial of what was achieved in mental hospitals of 50 or more years ago.

At the same time art therapy was developing strongly at Warlingham. This again was in line with current trends, and T.P. Rees was a great man for introducing the latest innovations into his hospital. The impetus came from the English painter Adrian Hill, who had seen the beneficial effects of art therapy and the exhibition of pictures in the sanatorium for tuberculosis at Midhurst before the war. Rees took up the idea; he appointed no less than three young female artists for whom these part-time appointments allowed them to continue with their rather precarious studio work. The growth of art and music in the hospital marked the first steps in integrating the two hospital cultures. It happened quite unconsciously and resonated with my own feelings.

From the beginning of my career in psychiatry I sought to obliterate the image of the mentally ill as an alien race. It began when I was seven or eight years old. Out driving with my mother we would sometimes pass the great asylums at Epsom and see lines of patients being escorted on a walk. Mother would remark on their 'queerness' and air her views on the hereditary nature of insanity, then current. From my first days at Warlingham I remember trying to relate to every patient as if there was no difference between them and any other variety of patient. Together with Erica Chance, a social worker with considerable group experience, I formed a mixed group of psychotic and neurotic patients. There were originally 12 patients, both men and women, including one epileptic patient. My notes on this group reveal the degree to which the psychotic patient is sensitive to revealing his psychotic ideas. Miss S., for example, claimed that she suffered from 'nervous exhaustion', suggesting that some unknown force had sapped her will. Pressed by the group she revealed that she believed her illness had been brought on by 'unseen forces'. Miss D. I noted was 'very hesitant and diffident and appeared to have difficulty in getting out of the world of ideas'. My summary of this session was: 'It is important that psychotic statements should be understood...and dealt with by the group as a whole.'

My non-analytical colleagues regarded the utterances of psychotic patients as something to record in the notes and thus justify their continued detention in hospital. I saw them as priceless material in my search for an understanding of madness. None of the psychiatrists I questioned had any idea what was the difference between the fixed ideas of the delusional patient and those fears to which we all fall prey, but which we put aside by rational thought or proof. Perhaps there was no difference, perhaps good and evil were the same. Fifty years later, I realise that what I was trying to do was to reconcile the opposites in myself. Jung himself warned of the dangers and tension associated with the process, but nevertheless he embarked on it himself in the seven years from 1913 to 1920 when he was exploring his own unconscious. Although I commenced a personal analysis in 1948, the quest for this reconciliation has been projected into my work for the rest of my life. I explored it in a long see-saw of alternating interest between neurosis and psychosis; between drug therapy and psychotherapy; by attempting to bring the 'two psychiatries' general and psychodynamic together; and in attaching a spiritual or religious dimension to my understanding of the patient. The tension could not continue forever, and I like to think that eventually I have understood enough about the opposites and about good and evil to be able to come down firmly on one side. It is the side of striving to understand every patient in dynamic terms, or perhaps I should say, understanding the human condition at every level.

The interesting thing about those beginning years was that no one said: 'This is what you should be doing, this is where you should look'. It is true that T.P. Rees urged, and even instructed, me to set up various projects, such as opening a club in Croydon for ex-patients and outpatients, but the way I set about these was my own. In 1948 I started a group for the female patients receiving deep insulin treatment. This treatment was invented by Dr Manfred Sakel at the Lichterfeld Hospital in Berlin in 1927, and fully developed in Vienna. It is said that he became convinced that the problems of mental disorders must be approached by medical means as well as psychological. Sakel (1954) said that the rationale for the treatment lay in its ability to 'overstimulate the vagus system', which antagonised 'the stress-defensive mechanism of the adreno-cortical system' (p.262). He added that the therapist was of course free to pursue his own therapeutic regime with his patient at the same time. The latter was clearly forgotten, and I think it likely that outside Vienna, deep insulin treatment was regarded in the same light as elec-tro-convulsive therapy (ECT) - namely, as a purely physical treatment. Sakel had initially reported a recovery rate of an astonishing 86 per cent, but this had come down to 12–14 per cent in the USA by 1939. Nevertheless its use continued until the mid-1950s in the UK and probably longer elsewhere.

It was here, in this group of patients receiving deep insulin treatment, that I learned something about schizophrenia from the inside. It was as seductive and exciting as my excursions into the heavens with my telescope had been, 20 years earlier. The beauty and the mystery of the star-filled sky at night was balanced by its inaccessibility, the enormity of unimaginable distances, and its mystery. The heavens were inhabited by ancient gods and mythical beings, and by the strange potential of the twelve signs of the zodiac. It was here that I came close to Jung and his studies of alchemy, which took me to the heart of the world of the opposites and of transformation. This is the world inhabited by the schizophrenic patient. During my first year in psychiatry I was puzzled by the nature of fixed delusional states, and gradually realised that the delusions were impervious to reality because my kind of reality simply did not exist for the patient. If it did, it was split off and belonged to another self. One of the patients in a long-stay ward believed herself to be an early British queen. She was indeed a queen in her ward, making tea and being pleasant to favoured people. Those rash enough to call her by her real name threw her into a violent temper, and she would shout, 'That's not me, that's someone else I hate.' In that same year I came across a man who believed there was a time bomb under his bed. Nurses could carry away imaginary bombs, doctors would reassure him, but his belief remained as strong as ever.

In my group of deep insulin therapy patients I began to learn what lay behind some of these delusional beliefs. In the period of recovery from coma and for an hour or two afterwards, when the patients were being cared for and nursed, they felt secure enough to project and bring alive their psychotic conflicts. J.B. said that there were two men who worried her, one was there to help her and the other was hostile and unpleasant. She projected these images on to another patient, Audrey. She said: 'Audrey must have been influencing my unconscious. She is not Audrey, she is Aubrey, she is a man, I don't want her near me.' She re-iterated the idea of self-sacrifice, which I discovered was common in the material of this group; 'I do not want to come round [from coma], I want to die, I want to sacrifice myself so that the others can recover.' Audrey herself thought that she had been responsible for the death of Christ, and repeated J.B.'s wish; 'I am responsible for all the sins in the world. I want to die so that others can live.'

Subsequently, J.B. told me that she believed I had two brothers. 'One of them was murdered at the cycle shop and I knew beforehand it was going to happen – it was a kind of telepathy. You have another brother who works on the male side of the hospital.' The next day she equated coma with the unconscious. I asked her what her unconscious was like. 'It is evil and unpleasant. In it I find demons and the instincts. I have always tried to lift myself out of the pull of the lower instincts. My sister had a baby when she was 15. Another sister had to marry because she was going to have a child. I don't want that; I am too attractive and therefore a temptation to men whatever I do. It is quite easy for me to distinguish between reality and imagination. But a lot of people say that what to me is imagination is only fantasy. They say my ideas about telepathy are only imagination but I know they are real.' In this account I am reminded of the age-old myths of two brothers, sometimes twins. So often in these stories, one has to die, or he meets a violent end.

I was at the stage in my career when I viewed the group as contributing to my understanding of the psychotic process. It was a group of eight women and therefore also fed my need to relate to the female psyche. I did not at the time reflect much on the therapeutic value of the group itself, but I noted what happened. It was clear that I had introduced another dimension which helped the patients to value reality. After all, day by day for six or more weeks they were being plunged into what they variously believed was the unconscious, death, a demon world, or sometimes heaven. The recovery process consisted of being forced into the world of reality. One patient remarked that it would be terrible to have to undergo the treatment alone; it was the group which made it possible to face it. Another was having her insulin for the second time and wondered why she felt so differently about it this time. 'When I had it before I always came round easily and I never had any of these fears.' The group was a verbal process, and words are reality.

Mrs M. was a lady who believed she had been turned to marble. After 24 comas she came round saying 'I am not marble, not marble', repeated many times. She moved her joints and limbs to reassure herself that she was not marble. She felt her hair, 'there are one or two knots still left', then she found a lipstick and covered her lips with it, 'before it is too late', and 'to make me look human'. Then she looked at another patient and said, 'She has had a great tragedy in her life – I doubt if anyone has ever loved a man as she has, but she could not marry, insulin prevented it, it separated her from legal marriage, she could only live in a natural union not recognised by the law.' Then she withdrew the projection, 'I am in love, but I am not sure whether I am married, insulin may have unmarried me, but I am more in love than ever.'

After 30 comas she said, 'I feel that I am no longer married when I am on this treatment. The group and my husband are in antagonism, it is like being married to the group instead of to him.' Finally, after 45 comas, she ended insulin treatment. She then told me the following: 'My husband met a girl at the office and decided that she needed psychological treatment, he has never done anything like that before. He brought her home and they talked in one room while I sat in another. This was all right and I thought he was doing her a good turn. I was rather gay myself during the war while he was away, and had several boyfriends. Then he said he would have to take her away for the weekend, which he did and I was extremely unhappy. Not long after that I had my breakdown.' She felt cold towards him but felt she must preserve the marriage for the sake of their two children. I did not see her again, and she did not return to the hospital during the subsequent three years before I left. Her revelation at the end of treatment explained much, and I was left with the beginnings of an understanding, both how real-life events can throw someone into psychosis, and how much pleasanter the psychotic world of fantasy can be. I also learned what a terrifying place it can be.

J.B. ended therapy after 52 comas. By this time she seemed stuck. She reported to the group day after day that she still wished to die, saying that she wished she had died in coma. She still believed that there were Germans lurking in the hospital and she said she could not trust anyone. She then started psychoanalysis with William Shepley, but I have no notes as to the outcome. I reflect now that she was given a chance which few schizophrenic patients in an NHS hospital today are likely to get.

Here are the experiences of another insulin patient after 21 comas. She felt that she was the mother of the world, the eternal virgin. In order to accommodate this, her sexuality was lodged in her head, where it was guarded by a wolf.

> She feels that her head sexuality is getting larger and therefore out of control. She feels that the power of some instinctual force is about to be released. She has begun to experience a real hunger for food, and can eat without a sense of nausea and sickness. The instinctual force lies at the back of her head. Hitherto she has fed the guardian wolf with ideas, sometimes he has to be fed with material objects, in which case she undergoes a submission to him. Just as objects in the room become swallowed up, so consciousness may also disappear. The consequence of this possession by an instinctual force is that the eternal virgin mother becomes obscured or even obliterated. This has for long been her intuitive fear. The world of insulin coma she describes as hard, solid and metallic, lacking in feelings and somewhat horrific.

At a later date I learned more about the wolf. The patient had an intense antagonism towards her father, she disliked his intellectualism, and what she called his shadows, such as his moods, his unkindness and his cruelty. Although the wolf kept the image of her father at bay he was 'no friend of mine'. When she was four or five years old she used to frighten her sisters by calling out: 'I've got a wolf inside me.' Although this was a game, she really felt that the wolf was there. Perhaps, I thought, schizophrenic patients are born with thinner layers between the strata of the psyche.

I have presented this material in order to explain what I learned about the psychotic process, and how it helped me to understand and relate to the kind of world which the patient inhabited. The insulin group also provided me with some important material about group dynamics, which I will describe in an appropriate place. My notebooks on the subject cover the period from January 1948 until September 1949. January 1948 was the month when I had taken and passed the final part of the exam for the Diploma of Psychological Medicine, which was generally accepted as the post-graduate qualification in psychiatry prior to the creation of the Royal College of Psychiatrists in 1971. This freedom, after two years of intensive study, allowed me to start finding out what mental illness was really all about.

Even psychiatrists have a context, and although it had formerly been a profession which tended to work in monastic isolation, I could not do this, although it has its attractions. Uncle Jack had urged me with his passionate cry of 'Girls, girls, girls, you must have girls', and from the age of 17, I found myself in the company of a great many attractive and interesting young women. Medical school continued the process. There were plenty of pretty nurses, and even prettier physiotherapy students, all of whom, in those days, had come from similar backgrounds to my own. Many of my contemporaries married nurses. But there was, as always, only one girl for me, whom I met on a chance walk on Wimbledon Common with a friend in 1935. After a long and frustrating courtship we were married in 1941. Three months later I joined the RAF for five and a half years. Our first child was born in 1943, the second in 1945.

Before the war my wife and I had been playmates. We exchanged a lot of ideas, but, apart from brief flashes, I knew little about her inner life. At Warlingham my centre was the hospital and its people. In my dreams I lived in the hospital, and my home was on the periphery. My life was exciting, there was no lack of food for my hunger to learn and discover. Above all, I was incredibly busy. Evelyn was marooned in a place alien to her, and today I marvel that she was able to stick it out for the five years we were at Warlingham. January 1948, which was when my work with the insulin group began, marked the beginning of what was probably the worst winter of the 20th century. Warlingham is in the Surrey hills, and the temperature did not rise above freezing for three months, snow lay deep and gradually turned to ice. The country was deeply impoverished by the war and had no reserves. Coal could not be moved, and for several weeks there was only electricity for an hour in the morning, two hours at midday, and for the same time in the evening. The hospital had its own generators and thus created an artificial oasis of apparent plenty and comfort in a frozen desert. It was a good metaphor for the schizophrenic state with its rich inner world of fantasy surrounded by the bleak reality of everyday life. And it was my experience of this inner world which set me on fire. Evelyn and I had lost what we had of that flame, and never regained it except for a few fleeting weeks when our marriage was beyond recall. But that was years later, and until Warlingham I had experienced the inner world of a woman only once, and she and I parted with great sadness when I left the RAF. We have never met since, but Louise will never be forgotten.

As a child I spent a lot of time looking, either looking through my telescope, or observing the weather, or just noticing things. My work as a physiologist in the RAF started with work on respiration at high altitudes and continued with work on night vision and on day-time visual acuity. I continued to build another span of this bridge at Warlingham with my interest in art therapy and art education, and at the level of metaphor, with insight, the study of dreams, including my own, and in 'visualising' the inner world of the patient. At a more objective level, I became interested in the way schizophrenic patients saw their external world as well as its inner manifestations. If you sit in a completely dark room and look at a pin-point light it appears to wander, and the pattern of its wandering can be mapped. My colleague Dennis Scott and I set up just such an experiment with the object of investigating whether there was any difference between the two eyes in the way schizophrenic patients experienced the behaviour of the light.

Here is one patient's account:

> It was red with the left eye as if someone had made a rectangular daub of red paint over the light. The bulb was faintly visible. The light made horizontal undulating movements to the left. There was a struggle in my mind to reach the light, the task was too difficult to perform. The light with the right eye looked clear and was fairly steady.

Two weeks later the square of light in the left eye appeared hard and glassy, while three days after this the light had returned to what I had observed when treatment began, ascending with the left eye, and fairly stationary with the right. She felt that the left side of her body had become dead and she had a sensation that a different eye had been grafted on to her which was harder and glassier than her own one.

I do not recall that we reached any striking conclusions from these experiments, but we did establish that there is a connection between the way we see objects and our mood which in turn reflects our psychic state. Some ophthalmologists have recognised their links with psychodynamics. Philip Inman, for example, who was still practising in Portsmouth at the age of 90 (1967), firmly believed that many who suffered from a stye, known medically as *hordeoleum* because of its being like a grain of barley, a fertility symbol, were associated with some act of generation, usually pregnancy. While writing this chapter I developed a stye, unusual for me. My wife said 'Are you pregnant?', and then I realised that we were two days away from the birth of a new century and a new millennium, a powerful event. The exchanges between body and mind are more subtle and varied than we sometimes care to acknowledge.

Today I still have a telescope, which I use when it is possible to avoid the pollution of man-made light. I also still have Uncle Jack's microscope, which I use less often. The eye which I use increasingly is the 'mind's eye', that wonderful organ which scans our dreams, paints pictures for our imagination, and reflects the events of the past. Some of these may have happened a few minutes, days or weeks ago; others, like those at Warlingham when the psychiatric world was young for me, are now long past. Above all, the mind's eye is about insight, that ability not only to stand back and see oneself objectively, but to make hitherto unrecognised connections. The schizophrenic patient, I discovered, is disconnected. The patient above who observed the wandering light had a disconnected appearance between her two eyes. The new eye on her left side was artificial, like a glass eye, and did not belong to her. After insulin therapy she was in analysis with me until I moved, when I referred her to a Jungian analyst, but I never knew the outcome.

One of the insulin patients told me that when she was first ill she felt that her soul had left her body and that she was unable to recall it. Hence she had lost all feeling, life was not worth living and she tried to end it unsuccessfully. She believed that an intervention by a higher power had saved her from death. After two insulin comas she experienced her soul re-entering her body, since when she had felt very well. She ended treatment and left hospital, I saw her once subsequently, when she had attempted suicide again and thought she was an angel. She was not my patient and I reflect now that it is sad that her initial change, when she got her soul back, was not followed up by psychotherapy. If this had happened, the experience of regaining her soul would have become integrated into her psyche.

It was patients who presented me with material like this that convinced me that I was right to follow Jung rather than Freud. At that stage I was quite violently opposed to Freud, complaining that he operated by a system of fixed symbolism, and that his methods were reductive and lacked all spirituality. But I was never happy with my feelings of antagonism, which went against my life-long desire to build bridges. Fortunately, time has done this for me, as there is now an understanding between the two schools which was unthinkable even 20 years ago. Nevertheless, as a medical staff we were a friendly lot and always continued a dialogue on our different viewpoints. I believe it was my fate to be drawn to what might be called the Jungian way. So much in my early life; my father's concern with the mysterious and the otherworldly, my interest in the mythological aspects of dreams, my desire to explore the far reaches of space, all resonate in that direction. In my last year at school a friend and I decided to revive a student journal called the *Science Magazine*, which we were successful in doing. I contributed an article on alchemy to the first issue. Unfortunately the text has been lost, but I know there was a reference to the Rosicrucians which would no doubt have warmed Jung's heart. The fact that I met a Jungian analyst at Warlingham, and that so many of the staff resonated to Jungian ideas, seemed to me to be heaven-sent. I have never become an orthodox Jungian, if there is such a person, but I have always understood what he meant, and tried to incorporate his meaning into my style of therapy.

During the Warlingham years I rediscovered my ability to write. The titles of some of the surviving papers will give a brief indication of the range of my interests which helped to shape the kind of psychiatrist I have eventually become.

I never published my material from the female insulin room, largely because Dennis Scott (1950) published a similar paper based on male patients which included some material from my own observations. The paper which I read at the tenth anniversary meeting of the use of insulin coma treatment in England is titled 'The psychology of insulin coma treatment' (1950), and remains extant. I have a large amount of material derived from this now almost forgotten era of psychiatry, and I learned a great deal. For example, after a detailed account of the progress of a male patient, I note that he was re-admitted to hospital in 1951. The social worker's report contains two significant remarks: 'His psychosis is closely related to his family situation', thus anticipating the work of Wing and others more than 20 years later (see Wing 1923 and Wing and Brown 1970), and, 'He says that when he is psychotic that is something more akin to his real nature, and that treatment brings him back to a state of normality which, however, is distasteful to him.' Here lies the source of a great divide. Psychodynamically, he is in greatest need of help when he is 'well'. The medical model demands that he be treated vigorously when he is 'ill', and discards him as soon as he is 'well'.

In 1948 the First International Congress on Mental Health was held in London. The professional staff of the hospital were invited to prepare a joint study on 'Family Problems and Mental Health'. Most of the medical staff, the social workers and the psychologist contributed. A group of eight patients was convened which met three times and their views were incorporated in the study. My own contribution was 'Family problems and psychological disturbance: The problem of extra-marital relationships'. While compiling it I sought the views of my patients at the Good Companions Club in Croydon. The problems of war-time marriages and the relationships occasioned by long separation occurred frequently in the case notes of our patients at that time. My choice of title no doubt reflected some of my own pre-occupations. My study was based on an examination of the notes of 179 male patients who were admitted to Warlingham during 1948.

Physical treatments were at the height of their popularity during my time at Warlingham. I conducted a study which was incomplete and which was designed to compare the outcome of patients admitted during 1926–1930 with those admitted during 1946–1950. I discovered that almost as many patients diagnosed as suffering from melancholia recovered in the earlier series as in the later one. All patients diagnosed as 'mania' recovered in the 1926 series, while 17 out of 31 patients suffering from schizophrenia recovered. Despite the flaws in the study, it is enough to dispel the myth that patients went into mental hospitals never to return.

I extended the insulin studies to ECT, and this was published in the *Journal of Mental Science* in 1950. It was another attempt to unite the physical with the psychodynamic.

I was particularly interested in the social aspects of mental illness and in the social relationships between group members. Together with Erica Chance, I compared the social structure of an in-patient group, an out-patient group and a youth club (1948). The youth club was situated on the New Addington housing estate, a suburb of Croydon which had been the pre-war brainchild of Henry Boot as a means of re-housing families from the slums of the East End of London. The result was a dismal wilderness. I never managed to complete my social and psychiatric study of the estate, but in the process I was persuaded to join the local general practitioner in judging a baby show. Over 90 babies were entered and we worked meticulously to get it right. However, we were nearly lynched by the mothers afterwards who were convinced that we had awarded the prize to the wrong baby. We both said, 'Never again!'

The out-patient group in the above study comprised some of those who attended the Good Companions Club. I wrote up the work and dynamics of the club more fully in 1951. My comparative work with the three groups had shown the extent to which psychiatric patients, particularly those who had been in hospital, lacked social skills. There can be no doubt that the club, with its many activities, greatly assisted in their creation or restoration.

There exists a group of papers on topics of lesser interest which give some idea of the range of my interests. I talked to social workers in Croydon about group therapy; also to hospital librarians on 'The approach to the patient', about which, in their own field, they knew more than I did. There is a collection of papers on various aspects of group therapy written by several members of the staff (Sandison *et al.* 1950). Another file gives an account of all the group and recreational activities existing in 1950 at Warlingham Park Hospital and in the Croydon Mental Health Service. I visited the Peckham Health Centre, where Dr Scott Williamson had, before the war, set up a family-orientated centre which was probably the first organised attempt to practice holistic medicine, and which marked the beginnings of family therapy.

Warlingham was noted for the interesting people that Percy Rees picked out to work there for a few months. Among these was Dr Samiran Banerjee, President of the Indian Psychotherapeutic Association. Banerjee decided that the patients at Warlingham, despite extensive and imaginative programmes of occupational therapy, were very institutionalised. In one sense he was right. On the other hand there is no doubt in my mind that there were a significant number of people in society who were happiest in the care of a well-run, imaginative and liberal hospital. This is certainly no less true today. Banerjee brought what he called a programme of 'activity therapy'. I think it was of more theoretical than practical use, but the patients enjoyed it, and he stimulated our thinking. Banerjee appeared again when he came to Powick Hospital in 1952, bringing the roots of the Indian shrub *Rauwolfia serpentina*.

In 1951, I had been associated with Warlingham Park for five years. My quest to understand the feminine psyche had reached the stage of courtship. Jung said that he talked to his anima for ten years before they reached any kind of mutual understanding. I had just concluded three years in analysis, and had many more years to go before I knew myself. But my close contact with many patients had taught me a lot about what it is like to be mentally ill. At the DPM course at the Maudsley Hospital I had learned to distrust systems of classification and diagnosis. I joined a group at the Tavistock Clinic run by Dr Elliott Jacques. It was a mixed group whose members included John Rickman, the distinguished Freudian analyst, some staff from the Tavistock, with myself and some students in various disciplines. I learned among other things how reluctant analysts were to disclose anything personal about themselves. For six months I spent one afternoon a week under the distinguished neurologist Wooster Drought. I gained a working knowledge of the subject, of which I was very glad when doctors referred patients for a psychiatric opinion whose symptoms turned out to be the result of a neurological disorder. I certainly learned a lot from Rees about how to run a large institution, and he taught me a lot about the doctor–patient relationship and transference problems. Above all he allowed me to develop my own way and to make my own mistakes.

Rees, and my peers, thought that I was ready to apply for consultant posts. The hospital had been my home, it felt more secure than any other place I had inhabited. Fate had it that I was appointed consultant psychiatrist at Powick Hospital, Worcestershire, and I left Warlingham to take up the appointment in September 1951. As I came down the stairs from the medical common room for the last time I shed a tear; I was truly leaving home.

CHAPTER 2

In Search of a Model, 1.
WORCESTER 1951–1964

I arrived at Powick Hospital, 4 miles from Worcester, early in September. The amenities were bleak in the extreme compared with Warlingham. The hospital had been built in 1852 for 200 patients. The wards were in two wings on either side of the medical superintendent's house. This house was now offices for medical staff on the ground floor, and residents' quarters above. Three-quarters of this ground-floor space was taken by the medical superintendent, Arthur Spencer, the hospital secretary and Spencer's secretary, a dismal sort of man who tried hard but whose abilities were limited. The remaining room was gloomily furnished with a large table and a few uncomfortable chairs. Arthur and I were the only consultants, and two assistant doctors completed the medical staff. There were nearly 1000 patients, 400 of whom were living in the four large wards of the 'annexe', built in the 1890s.

I discovered that the heating system was almost defunct, that many of the internal telephones did not work, and that the hospital was deeply impoverished in every department. Spencer suggested that he would look after the administration and that I should run the clinical side of the hospital. This suited me well, as he had a difficult committee, while the Regional Board in Birmingham needed a lot of convincing that Powick was worthwhile supporting. This state of affairs had been allowed to develop by the previous medical superintendent, Dr Fenton. An Edinburgh graduate, he was appointed Assistant Medical Officer in 1907, and died in 1950, having spent 43 years at Powick. He practised the utmost economy, and Powick became the cheapest hospital in the country. According to Hall (1989), under his jurisdiction, 'The asylum stopped being a hospital, and became a kingdom over which the medical superintendent held sway, managing it with justice, economy and administration, that is with managerial rather than clinical skills' (personal communication).

On that first morning in September, I was unaware of most of this history. I had scarcely hung my coat up before Dr Gwen Hobart came in, introduced herself and asked me to come to the ward immediately where a patient was in *status epilepticus*, a potentially life-threatening condition. I suddenly became aware that I was now a consultant, this was my responsibility, there was no one else. The patient turned out, as it happened, to be in a state of hysterical stupor, and subsequently I did a lot of psychotherapeutic work with her. As I went round the wards, I saw the effects of years of neglect and deprivation, and much of my work for that first winter was devoted to treating the effects of the cold and a poor diet.

Spencer and I spent the next year re-organising the hospital, and I believe it was during that time that we laid the foundations for it to become the first-class clinical unit which it achieved in the years 1958 to the mid-1960s. It was then that the hospital fell victim to its own success. The Minister of Health of the day decided that Powick and Worcestershire should be the 'test bed' for the proposed programme for the closure of mental hospitals and their replacement by 'community care'. As a matter of history, I left the hospital in 1964, Arthur Spencer retired in 1972, and the hospital ceased to admit patients in 1978. Another 'centre of excellence' had been dismantled for ever.

I had left what might be called the London scene because I wanted to develop my own ideas and not be part of someone else's domain. The region had some romantic associations which have always drawn me to places. The City of Worcester, lying on the River Severn, was ancient border country. The running stream of the river sang the lines of *The Shropshire Lad*, while the three great cathedrals, Worcester, Gloucester and Hereford, formed an ecclesiastical triangle redolent with memories of visits with my father in the far-off days when he was working with Ancient Monuments.

There was even a sense of romance about Powick Hospital. It had been built on 552 acres of ancient farmland known as White Chimneys. That name was written on the death certificate of every patient who died in the hospital, and this was still the practice in my time. From its opening in 1853 until Edwardian times it seems to have been a happy place. It was largely a self-sufficient village, and many patients were employed in its departments. Indeed, the first group of nursing attendants were all artisans, tailors, shoemakers, bakers, butchers and carpenters. The patients were included in many activities. In 1862 the head male attendant was married in the hospital, and a ball was held in the laundry, where upwards of 150 patients were feasted with plum cake and gin punch, and dancing took place from 7 until 11.30 in the evening. Edward Elgar had a long association with the hospital, being appointed bandmaster there in 1879. From that time until the 1940s every male nurse appointed had to be able to play a musical instrument.

Under the dead hand of Fentonism the patients and staff had been firmly regimented and nearly all the life and romance had gone from the hospital. On my first day I remember noticing the old chapel, a small architectural gem in a hollow of ground above the cricket field. It was used as a store, and a sort of Victorian barn attached to the main building had been built to the glory of God when the hospital was enlarged in the 1890s.

I can tease out the romance of Powick today, the reality at the time was a hard demanding clinical world. My dreams indicate that I had been the subject of much personal and clinical inflation before I left Warlingham. In 1950 I dreamt that I was present at the royal birth. Shortly afterwards I received a call from the palace as the Princess was threatened with puerperal psychosis. I cannot understand why I have been chosen, but learned that the Princess, in her delirium, spelt out my name. From these dreams my descent into reality begins. About the time I went to Powick I dreamt that I was in a room with six beautiful girls. This dissolves and there is only my wife Evelyn and myself, living in a tiny garret, where we are poor and I am ill. There is a beautiful gilded mirror on the wall, but its reflection is confused and disorientating. The poverty of our relationship is again reflected in a dream in which I am going home, but as I go the journey becomes ever more drab and dull. She is at home, lying cold and ill; we are starving. These dreams touch me today with a huge sense of tragedy that I ignored at the time. I recorded only these two dreams in 1951, and then there is silence until 1953.

I spent the first year, until September 1952, getting the hospital on its feet as a valid place to accept and treat patients. The staff was increased in almost every department, empty wards were reopened as admission units, clinical teams were created, out-patient clinics opened up. Everything, from the most basic items of clothing, diet and patient well-being, was looked at and up-graded. Psycho-therapy was gingerly introduced. Here there was a huge cultural gap to bridge, as I discovered that, for many years, no female patient had been interviewed by a doctor without the presence of a nurse. A process had been started which was to lead to the hospital becoming a centre of clinical excellence and internationally known within another six years. Meanwhile, at the end of that first year, I set off on a study tour of Swiss mental hospitals organised by Dr Isobel Wilson. It was a journey into the unknown, but it was to have far-reaching consequences both for me and for the lives of many future patients. The Sandoz laboratories in Basel and the Burghölzli Hospital in Zurich were among the first places we visited, and both changed the direction of my professional life.

Two visits to the Sandoz laboratories in Basel gave me my first sight of the work being done there on the ergot derivative known as Lysergic Acid Diethylamide (LSD). I met Drs Cerletti and Bircher, and on the second visit, Albert Hofmann himself, who synthesised the drug in 1938. A world of extensive research, unknown to me until then, was about to open. Bircher had also been working on the rauwolfia alkaloids, to which I had recently been introduced in England following the arrival at Powick of my old colleague Dr Samiran Banerjee. The latter had brought a parcel of the roots of the shrub *Rauwolfia serpentina benz*. That is another story which comes later.

I was tremendously excited by the work going on at Sandoz. Hofmann is a chemist, and, in 1942, five years after his initial synthesis of LSD, he was moved, by whatever forces is impossible to know, to re-examine his discovery. He wrote (1983):

> Yet I could not forget the relatively uninteresting LSD-25. A peculiar presentiment – the feeling that this substance could possess properties other than those established in the first investigations – induced me, 5 years after the first synthesis, to produce LSD-25 once again so that a sample could be given to the pharmacological department for further tests. (p.14)

As far as I can discover, Hofmann had displayed no special interest in those hallucinogenic compounds which were already known. Chief among these was mescaline. There was a flurry of articles in the medical press and elsewhere between 1896 and 1927, with which the names of Havelock Ellis, Lewin, Mooney, Mitchell and Prentiss among others are associated. Their work is well documented by Klüver (1928). In all this work the hallucinations, sensory changes and disturbed thought patterns are described in detail, but no parallel is drawn between the optical events and the 'inner life' of the subject. One subject who experienced a fretwork design attributed this to changes of sensory physiology, while another considered the same experience as not only of cosmic significance, but as the cosmos itself. This is described by Klüver as 'certainly an interesting contribution to the psychology of these subjects'.

Use of mescaline and LSD in the 1950s

Interest in mescaline continued to live on and was revived in the early 1950s, largely through Aldous Huxley's self-experiments (1954). Huxley's life goal seems to have been a search for the otherworldly, the mystical and the unattainable. He did not see mescaline as contributing to his personal development, but as an envious attempt to become a mystic, if only for a brief period: '…that, by taking the appropriate drug, I might be able to know, from the inside, what the visionary, the medium, even the mystic, were talking about … From what I had read of the mescaline experience I was convinced in advance that the drug would admit me, at least for a few hours, into the kind of world described by Blake and Æ' (p.9). (Æ: George William Russell (1867–1935). Author of *The Divine Vision* (1904) and volumes of mystical poetry.)

A number of people in the UK had taken mescaline during the 1950s. They were limited to journalists, members of Parliament, authors, artists and doctors.

This is very similar to the range of people who had taken the drug at an earlier period. It was still possible, but only just, to contain the use of hallucinogenic drugs to the consulting room and a small group of literati and intelligentsia. In less than ten years we would be on the edge of an explosion of hallucinogenic drug use.

Hofmann's discovery of the clinical properties of LSD

I think it unlikely that Hofmann was aware of the earlier work with hallucinogens when he resynthesised LSD in 1943. What happened when he did so and accidentally ingested a minute amount of the substance is related in an account of early work with LSD by Stoll (1947). Hofmann reported:

> Last Friday, 16 April, I had to stop work in the laboratory in the middle of the afternoon and had to go home as I was overcome with a strange restlessness and a slight dizziness. At home I went to bed and sank into a not unpleasant intoxicated state marked by the most stimulating effect on my imagination. In this drowsy state with my eyes closed (I found the daylight unpleasantly bright) fantastic pictures of extraordinary vividness and an intense kaleidoscopic interplay of colours forced themselves upon me without interval. After about two hours this condition gradually disappeared.
>
> On that Friday another extraordinary substance had been used in the laboratory, d-lysergic acid diethylamide … I had just succeeded in getting the d-lysergic acid diethylamide as a well crystallising tartrate, readily soluble in water. I could not, however, explain in what way I could have been affected by a sufficiently large quantity of the substance to produce the above mentioned syndrome … But I wanted to get to the bottom of this and I decided to experiment on myself with the crystallised d-lysergic acid diethylamide tartrate. (p.2)

It was here that Hofmann showed that he was more than a chemist. Already his innate intuition and desire to find the essence of things had been fuelled by the fascination and seduction of the phenomenon he had observed in himself. A few days after his original discovery he took 250 microgrammes (μg) in a watery solution:

> I asked my assistant to take me home as I believed it would take the same course as it did last Friday. But on the way home on my bicycle it was obvious that the symptoms were stronger than the first time. It was an effort to speak clearly and my vision was blurred and distorted like the image in a distorting mirror. I had a feeling that I was not moving although my assistant told me that we cycled at a good speed. (p.2)

All the manifestations of the drugs action were subjective. A doctor was called who 'found the pulse weak but otherwise the bodily functions were normal' (p.2).

Hofmann recalled that he could remember every detail of the experience with the greatest clarity. He wrote to Professor Stoll and Professor Rothlin about his findings, and both were astonished that so minute a quantity of LSD could have produced such a powerful effect. Displaying the same spirit of enquiry that Hofmann had shown, Professor Rothlin and two of his colleagues all took LSD, but used only one-third of the dose taken by Hofmann. Even so, 'the effects were still extremely impressive and quite fantastic. All doubts about the statements in my report were eliminated' (Hofmann 1983, p.21).

Hofmann and his colleagues then set up a programme of psychological and physiological research. LSD was given on a total of 49 occasions to 11 adult men and 5 adult women, mostly laboratory workers and students. Many measurements were made on these dedicated volunteers, and the results appear in Stoll's paper after the description of Hofmann's original experiment. Some of the observations made by the subjects foreshadowed the future possibilities of the use of LSD in psychiatry:

> I can watch myself all the time as in a mirror and realise my faults and mental inadequacies.

Another subject said that LSD had made her think of 'things better left forgotten'. Several wished to 'let go' emotionally, but felt ashamed to do so. These feelings reflect the setting, which was a strict laboratory one in Switzerland, where people were expected to behave properly. It should be noted that the subjects in these early experiments were uncontaminated by any expectations of the likely effects of LSD. In this they were unique. All subsequent work suffered from the possibility that the patients', and indeed the therapists', expectations could distort the patient's own perceptions. This was a view which I sometimes heard, and which some sceptical psychiatrists subscribed to. However, once you have sat for some time with a patient in the throes of an intense psychic experience under LSD such doubts disappear.

Hofmann then went to the Burghölzli Hospital, where he gave LSD on 20 occasions to 3 male and 3 female schizophrenic patients. The results, as may be expected, were inconclusive. Hofmann did not follow up this work immediately. In 1956 he took part in work which was being done in Czechoslovakia with patients.

I left Sandoz with Stoll's paper describing the work just quoted, with some work by Professor Mayer-Gross in England which had just been published (1951) and the first paper on the clinical effects of LSD outside Switzerland, published by Busch and Johnson (1950). More significantly, I had with me a box containing 100 ampoules of LSD.

The other visit which took place a few days later was to the Burghölzli Hospital, Zurich, where we met Dr Manfred Bleuler, whose father, Eugen Bleuler, had transformed the hospital. He also introduced the term 'schizophrenia' to describe what had previously been known as dementia praecox. Here in Zurich I felt that I had come to the centre of the world, and I expected that the spirit of Jung would still be living on in the wards and corridors of the hospital. Jung joined the staff of the Burghölzli in December 1900, and was associated with the hospital for the next nine years. It was here that he did his seminal work on schizophrenia, and his book *The Psychology of Dementia Praecox* was published in 1908 (Jung 1960). Observing the fantasies and hallucinations of schizophrenics led to his formulation of the concept of the collective unconscious. His word association test, which I had used at Warlingham, was one of his tools for exploring his patient's psyche. Unlike most medical tests, it was a tool which he and his patient shared equally.

Manfred Bleuler had a deep respect for his father, in whose shadow he lived. Eugene was the first medical director who, being Swiss, spoke the Swiss German dialect. He said that he spent much time talking to his patients, particularly the schizophrenics, and became convinced that intellectual deterioration did not necessarily occur in these patients. He made what Manfred called heroic efforts to make contact with the lost patients, and had long interviews with many of them. He was called 'father' by the nurses and the patients, he was surgeon to the hospital, he looked after the children of the staff and banked the savings of the nursing staff. Manfred claimed that the concept of schizophrenia as a purely psychological condition lay at the core of modern psychiatry in Zurich. Despite Bleuler's confident assertions I did not see much evidence, either in Zurich or in Switzerland as a whole, that psychotherapy for psychotics was being practised. Although Bleuler mentioned that Jung had worked in the hospital he made little of it, and thus my dream of touching the hem of Jung's garment vanished. All this changed when we visited the Jung Institute, where we were met by Carl Meier, Jung himself being away in the mountains somewhere. Meier had taken over from Jung as director of the Institute, and had some interesting views.

He said he was very concerned about the change which he had observed in the English psyche since the end of the war. The Germans, he said, had always had a barren spirit, but the desert-like appearance and manifestation of the psyche in English minds was something new and unpleasant. He took a pessimistic view, saying that he did not know when we would regain it and that the loss might well be permanent. It was an interesting assessment, in the light of future history, made nearly 50 years ago. Some today might agree with his judgement, but we will have to wait several centuries before we can say for certain what is happening to the contemporary psyche now. Meier had a particular intuitive wisdom of his own, but he worried me. Two or three years later I visited the Jung clinic again, once more hoping to catch Jung at home, but he eluded me once more. Carl Meier was most generous, and gave up most of a day to my visit. By that time I was deeply engaged with therapy using LSD, and he warned me not to talk to Jung about it, as he was greatly opposed to its use. I noticed that Meier's desk was covered with piles of papers, each one weighed down by a large stone. It felt as if Meier himself was, like Sisyphus, labouring behind the weight of a large stone. I told him about a dream I had had recently in which the Queen and her mother had come to live in Worcester, and that the Queen Mother had become my own mother. I think Jung would have made something of this dream, but all Meier said was, 'Our patients in Switzerland also dream about your Queen.' He did, however, add that he believed that the young Queen fulfilled an anima role in dreams.

Carl Meier had many stories. He identified with all those regarded today as the 'underprivileged'. He would go into a long-stay ward and intuitively pick out a very lost patient whom he knew he could help. He said that sometimes, when such a patient recovered his grasp of reality, they would discuss how it had happened, and neither of them could say. He thought that his most interesting patients had been peasants and uneducated people. They would produce the most extraordinary material with an honesty and naivety which was uncomplicated by intellectual prejudice and education in the classics or history. He thought that the most interesting patient he had ever had was a Spanish Jew who could trace his family back to before the exile – namely, for over 2000 years. This patient had a series of what Meier called entirely primitive fantasies and dreams. Any attempt at interpretation of these left the patient entirely at a loss; he could not understand what was being said. It turned out that these dreams were in his own language, and that he was psychologically living in the period before the Jewish exile. He went on to talk about symptoms. At one time a great many peasant patients from the mountain districts came to see him, and he discovered that they were all interconnected. They all believed that Dr Meier had cured their symptoms, but Meier himself had been unaware that any of these patients had ever had any of the symptoms the others described. He thought that it was often desirable to leave the patient with his symptom as being the only thing of value which he possessed. We had a long discussion about transference, when he again reiterated his belief that in England what he called 'the spiritual forces in the people' were so lost and barren that the patient may project everything on to the analyst, who becomes the only spiritual force in the patient's world. I believe I was thinking of one of my own patients when I was discussing this, as my notes record Meier as commenting 'if the patient can project the spirit on to the therapist *she* must have it herself'. He urged me to 'hang on long enough, and she must find someone or somewhere on which to rest it in the end, and she must eventually find and realise it in herself'. If it was the patient I am thinking of, that is exactly what happened.

The Switzerland of 1952 was a place of gaiety and plenty. I linked up with two consultant colleagues, and we spent our evenings together enjoying good food, wine and conversation. After the drabness of England, still in the grip of rationing and austerity, it was a miracle. Not for over 13 years had we known anything like it, and we made the most of it. Our hosts were alive to our deprivations. Even the teetotal and abstemious Bleuler feasted us to capacity at a mountain restaurant, where the proprietor had killed a pig in our honour and Döle flowed freely. At Waldau in the Berne canton Professor Klaesi greeted us as 'the saviours of the world', and when we said we could only stay two days, he commented: 'What a pity, when I had planned to make you drunk for a week.' He did his best in the time available. The setting, the freedom from austerity, and the pleasures of civilised travel all combined to make the journey itself more important than some of its objectives. I learned much, but what touched me was the potential of the new substance, LSD.

In England, I was determined to set up a clinical programme using LSD as a tool to assist the growing level of psychotherapeutic work being practised at Powick. In this I received every possible help from Dr Harold Holgate, Sandoz's chief medical officer in London. Sandoz issued a detailed study of the history, properties and clinical effects of LSD in December 1951, which was updated in December 1952. Animal studies are followed by a résumé of the physiological effects on human volunteer subjects. These were minimal, but the subjective symptoms experienced after doses of the order of 20–100 microgrammes (μg) were wide ranging, varying greatly from person to person, and difficult to classify. The researchers of the day tried hard to equate the mental experiences of normal subjects with the known psychoses. Rinkel et al. (1952) distinguished a manic expansive reaction and a schizophrenic reaction with depersonalisation and hallucinations. Other researchers found that LSD reinforced existing characteristics producing a caricature of the subject. LSD was thought by Stoll (1947) and others to make it possible for the psychiatrist to study in himself some of the mental symptoms which he is called upon to analyse and treat in his patients. The opinion was expressed that LSD made patients more accessible to psychoanalysis by improving contact with the therapist and facilitating the recall of memories.

The work of Busch and Johnson (1950) has often been quoted in support of these ideas. However, the number of psychoneurotic patients (5) in their series (29 patients in all) scarcely justified some of their conclusions. They suggested that LSD facilitated communication with some very withdrawn patients, and that LSD might prove to be a new tool for shortening psychotherapy. Stoll's work (1947) was more convincing and his clinical description of the patients at the Burghölzli Hospital who received LSD is very detailed, as were the experiences of the volunteer subjects. There was as yet no theoretical basis for supposing that LSD could be used as a practical tool in combination with psychotherapy, but it was clear from the work already done that it produced a loosening of mental associations, that it facilitated the transference, and that forgotten and sometimes painful memories could be released. Mayer-Gross (1951), writing on his work with mescaline, had suggested that in cases of depersonalisation, subjecting the patient to a drug would itself intensify this symptom and that it 'would be justifiable to attempt the production of a severe mescaline intoxication in the hope that the depersonalisation may clear together with the other toxic symptoms of the drug' (p.320).

After discussion and consultation with my colleagues at Powick, and with the Professor of Psychiatry in Birmingham, I undertook the clinical use of LSD at Powick Hospital towards the end of 1952. The results were published two years later on the treatment of 36 patients (Sandison 1954; Sandison, Spencer and Whitelaw 1954).

LSD does not behave like any other drug in the pharmacopoeia. It produces its psychological effects in minute doses, the observable bodily changes are minimal. The effect varies not only from one person to another but in the same person on different occasions. It is not a drug in the specific sense of other remedies. I saw it as a tool for the promotion of psychotherapy, and I still maintain the same opinion. Today, when LSD is regarded by its protagonists as a 'recreational drug', it is difficult to understand the esoteric nature of this remarkable substance. Those of us who used it in clinical practice developed a reverence for its properties, rather as the shamans of old regarded their magical plants. Indeed, LSD belongs to the group of hallucinogenic substances which characterise many ancient healing cultures in South America and elsewhere. Some, such as mescaline and psilocybin, derived from a Mexican mushroom, are still in use today. I identified three distinct types of experience in the patients to whom we gave LSD:

1. Hallucinatory experiences of a dream-like nature, which I believed had their origin in the unconscious of the patient.

2. The reliving of forgotten personal memories.

3. The appearance of impersonal or collective unconscious images.

The following accounts from two patients will demonstrate the quantity and intensity of the experiences. Each image, each fantasy and each feeling is not only important to the patient, but must be explored by the therapist for it to be understood and integrated by the patient. Many accounts written by those who have taken LSD casually, or without analytical supervision, suggest that consciousness is bombarded with a succession of chaotic images. These are often described as horrific, and there is a sense of being overwhelmed. When patients took LSD and were carefully supervised, the visual images can be directed in the way that active imagination can direct fantasies. The process then becomes more like a cinematograph, portraying an orderly succession of events. Indeed some patients likened their LSD experience to being in a cinema. This view was echoed by a Jungian colleague, Margot Cutner (1959), who, by good fortune, elected to come to Worcester in 1952:

During three years work with LSD at a mental hospital…the writer noticed, more often than would be due to pure chance, that the material emerging under LSD, far from being chaotic, reveals, on the contrary, a definite relationship to the psychological needs of the patient at the moment of his taking the drug. (p.6)

The account given by one of my patients will illustrate this. She was a married woman, 29 years of age, born in Germany.

I began to see a face on the wall, it was a man with one eye and he had a moustache. He sometimes smiled at me cynically and sometimes looked very grim and threatening. I tried to connect him to something which had happened to me a long time ago. It was then that he got mixed up with Hitler and I saw nothing else but swastikas. For one brief moment it was my father's face. Then I remembered one man in particular; he was a German officer. Then I remembered the incident connected with that man.

The patient then described how this officer took her to his flat one evening and seduced her. She continued:

The thing that bothered me most under LSD was that I was forced against my will without showing the slightest resistance. As I pondered over this, Hitler appeared again and I saw the connection. He too, in a very subtle way, together with his powerful personality, made me do things against my will without my resisting. Then I had a feeling of falling down deeper and deeper and yet I felt detached just as if I was watching it all happen.

In the next LSD session the material seems to have no connection with any real incident in the patient's life.

There was a huge image of Hitler on the wall like a big shadow in which I could see many hostile faces. I wanted to get away from these hostile men and tried to hide in a corner. Then I saw skulls and crossbones on the wall and suddenly I felt the flesh falling off my bones and I was a skeleton, but I think only from the waist down. I remember my teeth falling out and when I tried to bite I was biting on my gums.

During several subsequent treatments the patient experienced similar occurrences of an unpleasant nature, seeing herself, for example, as a prostitute stabbed and lying in the gutter. She also became depressed and suicidal. The 10th treatment was described by her as follows:

There is tremendous confusion within me. There is no harmony. The muddled faces had terrific mouths and tried to swallow me up. I feel that they would swallow me up only as long as they were in such a muddle and it was therefore necessary to find order in this confusion. I then found that there was order in this confusion insofar as there were two sides to it each opposing the other and pulling in two directions. I tried to find out about the two parts and discovered that they must be the good and evil in me.

She then had this dream. In the beginning of the dream she meets her lover and feels very happy, but she cannot make love to him:

I tried to find out why I could not make love to him and suddenly something inside me said: 'Because you have not picked up the five heavy stones from the bottom of the sea. You did not do it for your parents either, that is why you could not love them.' I felt as if all my problems had been solved, at least I now know what I have to do.

In the next LSD session she decided to investigate this.

I feel I must overcome my fear and go to the bottom of the sea. Then I started going down, but under the water I met alligators who were eating me up and I could feel their teeth in my body. I went down under the water again and as I went deeper the fear grew less. I could see the stones, but now they were only four in number. It was as if the fifth had represented the fear which was now gone. With this stone gone I had a better view of the others. I came closer and closer and suddenly it was as if I was looking in a mirror. These four stones formed a face. I cannot describe its ugliness and horribleness. At the same time the face was beautiful. I could not say what piece was ugly and what was beautiful, for in it were both extremes completely merging and forming a whole. I felt that these were my anchors and on these I had to build up my personality. I

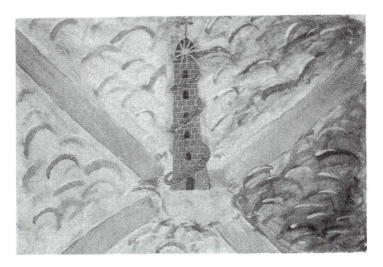

Figure 2.1 The patient under LSD visualises a crossroads, on which a lighthouse is erected in the next session

knew too that this was the same in all of us and everything alive. I had a feeling that what I had just seen was part of God.

She made several paintings of this sequence. The first painting is of a crossroads, which also represents the cross of Christ. In the next, a lighthouse is erected on the crossroads, with a serpent twined around it. Then comes the painting of the four stones. In their centre is a face which she said contained all the beauty and all

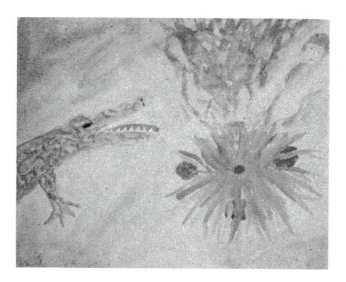

Figure 2.2 The patient dives down into the ocean to investigate the five stones. The alligator represents fear.

the ugliness in the world. In the next, the face had become transformed into a rich jewel, described by her as being beyond all price.

These images contain a great deal of archetypal material, which led me to believe that LSD opens up a high road to some of the deeper and collective aspects of the unconscious. In this they are identical with the dreams of some patients during the course of analysis. They are not an end in themselves, but they are indications that individuation is an attainable goal. Moreover, the objectification of the individuation process takes on a different, but universally recognisable, form for each individual. One might say that for the above patient the sea is a symbol for her mind, or her unconscious, and that the lighthouse and the stones are associated with the sea. The number five is an awkward one, but by discarding the fifth stone she achieves the satisfactory regularity and harmony of the four. Good and evil come together in the several ways she presented her material.

Another patient went through a similar process, but the icons are quite different. She was also a married woman, 26 years of age. She was in a very desperate state when she came to us. Her mother had died when she was young, her father was restless and psychopathic, her marriage had failed, and she had gradually severed all human ties until her only feeling was towards her dog. She suffered from night terrors and had an abnormally great fear of spiders. I took her on for psychotherapy, and after a few months she started LSD as an adjunct to the therapy. She re-experienced the night terror in which she cried out 'Oh, no', repeatedly, and soon came to realise that this was her response to her mother's death. On the first day she felt that she passed back through the whole of her life. At lunch her food appeared to turn into a dish of asparagus cooked by her mother. By tea-time she was a small child, keeping her food possessively to herself. Then she wished only to look at picture books and finally she lost her power of speech.

On the following day she had recovered her adult nature, but was filled with a great hunger 'I know not for what'. In the next LSD session the spider appeared, huge and menacing. There were continuous images of the spider and its four eyes: 'The spider never touches me but seems to want to enfold me and take me bodily, then I remember thinking that I myself was the spider.' A few sessions later this process had developed.

> I found myself inside a cell of my subconscious mind. It contained my spider, no longer alert and frightening and vivid, but tired, beaten and almost dead. It

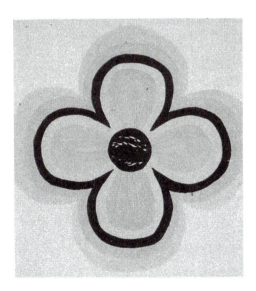

Figure 2.3 The final resolution of the spider into a flower-shaped mandala. The remnants of the spider are seen in the centre.

looked pathetic. With the spider there were thoughts and feelings and from these the conscious person, myself, had to learn a lesson. It was a most peculiar sensation. I found that my conscious self 'A' was speaking to my subconscious self 'B'. B was doing the teaching and A was learning, but it was also a two-way process.

She painted a picture of this situation, in which four circles fit together in a square. The fourth cell was larger and was the 'cell' of her mind referred to above. Finally, in a later experience, the spider, highly modified, lies in the centre of the four circles, now arranged like the petals of a flower. This is her mandala. This does not mean the end of the story. There was still a great deal of work to be done before she was able to integrate the creative power of the flower with four petals.

The third patient in this series was a young woman of 25 years of age. She had been engaged to several young men, but always reached a point where she became tormented with evil thoughts about them, sometimes that they were potential murderers. At one time she attempted to counteract these thoughts by taking an active part in the life of the Church, but found that her very worst thoughts would come to her in Church. There seemed to be no remedy, but 18 months of psycho-

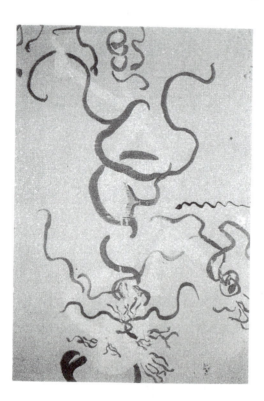

Figure 2.4 The serpents attached themselves to almost every part of her body

therapy had shown her the problem, but she saw no way of coming to terms with it. After her third session of LSD she wrote the following:

> I had the sensation of a snake curling up round me. I began to see serpents' faces all over the wall, and then I saw myself as a fat, pot-bellied snake slithering away to destruction. I realised that I was destroying myself. I was having a battle between life and death, it was a terrific struggle but life won … I told the doctor that there were snakes everywhere, and that I was in the middle of them. I discovered that I had had a dream like that when I was a child. He asked me what it represented and I said 'sex'. When discussing this I was right back as a small child with moving grass all round me and I could see snakes slithering through the grass. The whole atmosphere was as it had been during sexual incidents with boys when I was six or seven.

She then experienced herself as the devil and she saw her long pointed tail curled around me. It was one of those powerful moments which characterised LSD therapy, when it was all too easy to enter the patient's mythical world and thus lose one's ability to represent the one stable, sane point in the patient's experience. During the following night this patient woke up and reported:

> I had a sensation of watching myself. I was out of hell, standing on the brink and I was perfectly pure. I felt that I might be drawn back in again so I made myself run away. However, I was drawn back and I looked down into hell, and there was my snake still there in hell. I jumped back into hell and fell right into the snake's mouth and became the snake. Then I started the ascent out of hell, but it was a terrific struggle – I seemed to be carrying a huge weight but I kept struggling to get out. Then I felt the snake biting my tail – then I realised that I was biting my own tail and eating myself up. The struggle to get out of hell was too great and I thought that it wasn't such a bad place after all, so I curled up in hell and went to sleep.

Once again this was the beginning, rather than the end. Much had to be integrated which involved several months of psychotherapy, but the process had started. Here the redeeming symbols are the serpent and the uroboros, the tail-eater, regarded by Jung as a mandala symbol.

As time went on we established a blue-print for the effective use of LSD as a therapeutic tool. These principles were set out in our first paper in considerable detail, and would serve today if ever LSD again became available as a therapeutic tool (Sandison et al. 1954). Our method of working can be summarised in this statement: 'The treatment unit should be under the care of a psychiatrist who is thoroughly versed in the theory and practice of psychotherapy. His assistants should have a clear understanding of the principles of psychotherapy and case conferences should be held regularly' (p.504). We also laid down guidelines for staffing the unit, on the importance of frequent and clear communication between the medical and nursing staff, and on training of staff. We published the instructions given in writing to the nursing staff, which, among other matters, emphasised the importance of the after-care of the patient.

This paper generated both national and international interest in the possibilities of the use of LSD in psychiatry. It marked the end of an era. Before 1954 the media had taken scant interest in psychiatric treatments. There had been a good deal of coverage of the First International Conference in Psychiatry, held in London in 1948, some of which was irritatingly inaccurate, but its intention was factual. LSD provoked a more sensational reaction. Perhaps it was no surprise that journalists were fascinated by those who had experienced themselves as small children during therapy. One patient 'became a child of 5 or 6 years of age in the LSD experience. She felt that her clothes were huge, and when the doctor grasped her hand his hand seems large, as an adult's hand would to a child.' Hence LSD gained the reputation of being the 'Alice-in-Wonderland' drug. A journalist wrote in the *News Chronicle* (1953):

> 'This medicine,' the doctor said holding out a spoonful to the young woman, 'is going to make you live over again a day in your past. You are going to be a little girl again.'

Needless to say, we never made predictions of any kind to our patients as to what they might experience. Despite this unpromising start the writer advised caution:

> Although it seemed useful in uncovering repressed memories, the doctors indicate that it will never be given by any doctor simply because the patient thinks he or she would like to have it.

Curiously enough, I cannot find any such statement in our early papers on LSD therapy and from which I have already quoted. It seems that this astute journalist had already surmised that LSD produced such extraordinary changes in the psyche that the dissemination of this knowledge would lead to demands based on the 'everyone can have everything' principle.

The use of LSD in psychotherapy was a totally new approach to the problem of psychoneurosis and associated conditions. As with all new treatments in medicine we followed the established principles of the day. Having said that, I feel that no further defence of what we were doing is necessary. As a team, we shared our excitement and sense of discovery with the patients. I summarised this in the last paragraph of my first paper:

> The patients in the hospital group are all aware that LSD is a new drug for assisting the unconscious to reveal its secrets and one has been most encouraged by the help they have given in the work of investigating its uses. Many patients have assisted at clinical meetings by describing their experiences or actually having the treatment for the benefit of other doctors. My thanks are due to the many patients who have contributed to this work... (Sandison 1954, p.514)

This is reflected in comments made by a patient in 1957, concerning treatment she had had three years previously:

> In those days I think the doctors knew little more than the patients about it … Sometimes I could almost think I was in a test tube. I am sure the doctor suffered from wondering what was going to happen next and was he clever enough to deal with it…

> I think LSD was a wonderful opportunity and I would not have missed it for anything. I felt I had been given a chance so few people get to have contact with my innermost self, but I think also the drug can be dangerous.

This involvement of the patients in our own thinking became part of the therapeutic alliance. Without it, the patients might realistically have had fantasies of being part of a laboratory experiment.

Many patients expect that psychiatric treatments will take them back to some traumatic event in childhood, and that the exploration of this will be the 'cure'. It is, of course, an oversimplification based on some of Freud's ideas. Nevertheless, these discoveries can be very releasing. Here are two examples. The first patient was a young married woman with a great fear of sex. She could not contemplate pregnancy and she had a fear of hurting or killing children. She reported on a key session:

> My reaction to last Friday's treatment seemed to follow a different pattern. Instead of the usual feeling of mounting tension until a state of panic is reached, I remained quite calm, but when the reaction came it was sudden. Between spasms of difficult breathing I tried hard to think of a reason; slowly the feeling of someone behind me began to develop; there was only a wall behind me; nothing touched me and I saw no-one, it was only an atmosphere. During the next spasm the feeling of someone behind me was stronger. I began to feel anxious about my legs, it was an odd abstract anxiety … I felt under my pillow for a handkerchief, it wasn't a handkerchief, but a hand. I jumped up and looked behind me, but of course there was no-one there and it was my handkerchief that I held. I think it was about then that I realised that I was reliving an incident that occurred when I was quite small, on holiday at Bournemouth. I wondered if I had gone small and was not in the least surprised to see my hand and arm quite little, the size of a child of seven or eight. I don't remember feeling a different size, but when I looked I had shrunk. This was the first time I had gone small under treatment. It seemed to me that I was shopping with my mother in a large store in Bournemouth. She had walked on without my realising it and when I turned to speak to her I was alone and lost. I stayed where I was and turned to look at the counter beside me. Suddenly I felt someone behind me. I repressed an urge to cry out in case it was someone playing a joke. Although I do not know exactly what happened I think he must have put an arm round my throat. I was unable to turn

my head to see who it was. I was shocked to feel his hand on the inside of my thigh, but could only imagine he had chosen an odd way to take my purse.

My patient then described the interruption of this assault by a passer-by, the escape and capture of the man, his wild and insane appearance, his struggling wildly and his second and final escape.

A woman of 44 years of age had suffered from severe and obsessional fears since the death of her father three years previously. She reported after an LSD session as follows:

> I was icy cold, but found myself in a colour world again which dissolved into a fishing village which I knew ... I was sat in a deck chair. I held my sun-glasses and on the grass I could see my wide-brimmed hat, a book and my knitting bag. I can remember looking all round, seeing the cows quietly grazing, admiring the deep green of the grass, lifting my eyes to the sky, seeing the deep blue and the white-flecked clouds. My eyes travelled to the other side of the river. I was appreciating the beauty of everything. I then dropped my eyes and standing about four yards away was my father with his fishing rod in his hand. He turned round and smiled at me. I could see his face in vivid detail. Two or three yards away stood my husband but he was intent on fishing so I could only see him side-faced with an old sports jacket and a very battered trilby hat on and smoking a pipe. The sun was shining and the whole scene was peaceful and lovely. I returned to consciousness to find it snowing, but all the rest of that day and actually ever

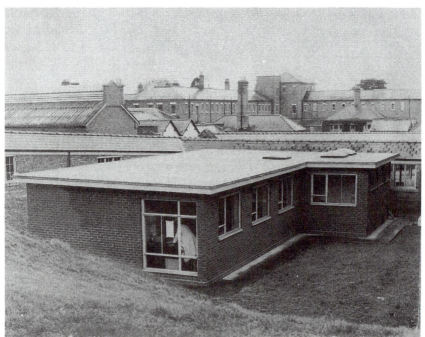

Figure 2.5 The purpose-built LSD unit, about 1960. Access from the main corridor behind.

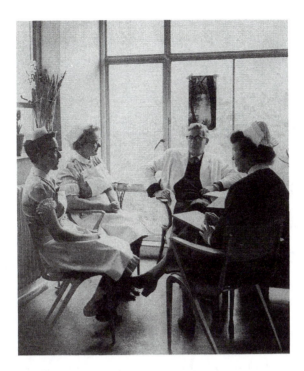

Figure 2.6 The author in conference with nursing staff of the LSD unit, 1960.

since, that picture has remained with me as something too precious to part with because my father had died just before my illness. That is three years ago this year, and owing to his illness we hadn't fished for some two years, but since I have been in this hospital I had forgotten that we had ever gone and yet it formed part of our summer weekend to spend the day fishing on Saturday or Sunday.

After the publication of our first two papers on LSD we made representations to the Regional Hospital Board for purpose-built premises to continue and develop the work. This materialised in the building, during 1955, of a unit known, rather unimaginatively, as 'The LSD Block'. It consisted of two rooms for the nurses, five rooms for the patients, and an area suitable for group meetings of either staff or patients. Each area was interconnected by a corridor. The rooms for the patients contained a couch, a chair, and a blackboard on the wall opposite the couch. This was much used by patients who wished to draw with chalks.

The setting up of the unit, and working with the intense experiences of my patients, gave me an entirely new focus. The process went some way towards fulfilling my dream of integrating traditional psychiatry with psychodynamics. What it actually achieved for me was a bringing together of my need to combine

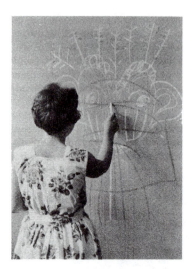

Figure 2.7 A patient drawing on the blackboard in her room during LSD therapy.
Photograph taken by N. MacKenzie

being a 'proper doctor' with my desire to be a healer of minds. Psychologically it was a development of the transitional phase which commenced in the insulin room at Warlingham. The latter consisted largely of observation, as I was not actively engaged in interacting with the patient's material psychodynamically. There was a sense of movement and drama about the LSD experience with which Uncle Jack's stories of medicine in Gallipoli, at the front in France and in the Shetland Isles had conditioned me to expect from the 'real' practice of medicine. This need on my part persisted for many years, and became partly split off when I intensified my interest in reproductive medicine and family planning, and acupuncture, in the 1970s.

This was a time of great professional activity. There is a long tradition of teaching in my family, and, with the growth of interest in LSD, I found myself much in demand from those hungry to learn about this new approach to psychiatric treatment. Most of the registrars at Powick were keen to work in the unit. Many visitors came, at first from the UK, later from many European countries, and USA, India, Canada, Australia and other commonwealth countries. In 1955, I was invited by The American Psychiatric Association to address a Round Table at their annual meeting. It was a momentous event, and to get there I decided to fulfil a dream of crossing the Atlantic by sea. The days of the great Atlantic liners were almost gone, and the thinking of the time was to combine a container ship with single-class passenger accommodation for about 70 people. Thus I set sail in the *Parthia*, 17,000 tons, on 30 April 1955. The sea was my first love. Coming from Shetland as I did the sea was by turns romantic, beautiful beyond compare, capable of changing to tempestuous fury in minutes, always to be revered, feared and deeply respected. The voyage should have taken seven days, it took ten. After four years of unremitting clinical work I abandoned myself to the pleasures of travel, of seeing no land for days on end, of good company and conversation and exquisite food. As we left the Mersey on a grey foggy morning the tolling of a bell-buoy had a mournful and eerie sound. It reminded me of those stories I had heard as a child of the water fairies who sang laments before a tragedy at sea. I was not disappointed, a severe storm in mid-Atlantic left us hove-to for three days. It was a frustrating delay but one which seized me with a flush of energy. I tore up the paper I had written for the conference and wrote a new one. I started to get the framework for a theme which afterwards I wrote into a novel, *Simon's Daughter*, published in 1984. In this Simon is a physiologist researching LSD. On his way to America he meets and has a brief affair with a married woman whose husband works in Canada. He does not meet his daughter who was born of their union for 14 years. Perhaps she was the daughter I never had. I was not looking for such an affair during that voyage. I was in love with LSD, for, as Simon said, it was the greatest love affair in the world.

The sea exacts a high price from those who love her, and so does LSD, as its history during the next 20 years amply demonstrated. The sea requires that those who sail on her do so with knowledge, respect and true love. LSD, like the sea, was prepared to destroy those who used it without full knowledge, or without respect or love.

Fortunately there were many who intuitively knew this. Although the psychoanalytical community was generally opposed to using LSD, there were some who did and who contributed greatly to its potential use. The Jungian analyst Margot Cutner, who joined the staff at Powick in 1955, observed that the material emerging under LSD, 'far from being chaotic, reveals, on the contrary, a definite relationship to the psychological needs of the patient at the moment of taking the drug' (Cutner 1959, p.6). She showed how self-regulatory processes in the unconscious facilitated the development of the patient by acting in a compensatory way to consciousness. In the same year Betty Eisner, of Los Angeles, had read a paper at a meeting in Rome expressing similar ideas (Eisner 1959). She worked in the Freudian tradition, but reached much the same conclusions as Cutner. Joyce Martin was a Freudian analyst who worked in private practice and at the Marlborough Day Hospital, London. She treated a series of patients: psychopathic personalities, obsessional states and homosexuals. Her paper (Martin 1962) reflects the wholly different way in which society and analysts held homosexuality from that of today. Astonishingly, she reported that seven of the twelve patients treated for this condition became heterosexually orientated. She followed up her patients for three and six years, and claimed that only one homosexual had 'relapsed slightly'.

They were euphoric years, but my enthusiasm stood up to the test when measured against the conservatism of institutions. In 1961 that long-established and august body The Royal Medico-Psychological Association (RMPA) devoted the whole of its February quarterly meeting to the use of hallucinogenic drugs in psychotherapy. It was most unusual, if not unique, for this three-day meeting to be devoted to a single topic. Furthermore, some of the speakers were from fields other than medicine or psychiatry, thus facilitating a development I had always hoped for at conferences on psychological medicine. It was a most stimulating event, with a high level of excellence from the contributors. Richard Crocket and I spent the next year editing the proceedings together with some valuable help from Alexander Walk (Crocket, Sandison and Walk 1963). The establishment continued to support an important and radical modification of psychotherapy which had, by the early 1960s, attained the status of a subspeciality. In 1962 I was invited to give the Maudsley Bequest Lecture at the RMPA, which I regarded as a further seal of approval from my own profession.

Therapy based on the Powick model was widely practised in the UK. In Denmark there were several centres promoted by the Danish analyst Thorkil Vangguaard, who had made a number of visits to Powick, and was, at that time at least, a good friend. LSD therapy was being practised in most of the major centres in Europe. In Czechoslovakia, Milosz Hausner had an excellent and innovative centre at Sadska, which he managed to keep going even after the Communist invasion in 1968. In Rome, Emilio Servadio, a training analyst, gave LSD to his trainees as a postscript to their analysis. His conclusions were very positive, although he remarked that the inclusion of this refinement imposed considerable demands on both analyst and trainee (Servadio 1964). Howard Whitaker, an analyst in Australia, reported on 100 cases treated using LSD as an adjunct to analysis (Whitaker 1964). Of course, a tremendous amount of work was being done in America, both North and South, and some of the analysts in Argentina reported on very large series. Without enlarging the list further, it will be evident that, for the space of nearly 15 years, psychotherapy enhanced by LSD was being practised on a scale which has never been exceeded. Numbers are not in themselves indicators of excellence or quality, but the era of serious and well-documented therapy must go down as an important event in medical history. Today, it is not so-judged, almost certainly owing to its misuse by some of its practitioners who were shipwrecked by LSD. I see them setting out like some inexperienced sailor convinced that his craft can face anything the sea can offer. One by one the governments of the world made LSD an illegal drug. Its effect on therapy was as if, following a few shipwrecks, the nations of the world had closed down all sea routes. There were other events stirring in my life, and, in 1964, I sought fresh field in Southampton. It marked the end of LSD therapy for me personally, but, as I shall show, the healer had turned into destroyer when LSD became freely available for street use in the early 1960s.

LSD was by no means my only focus of interest during the Powick years. It was a means of bringing together the physician and the mind healer in myself. I made several other excursions into the same territory, but LSD, measured by its benefit to patients, emerged the clear winner.

I have already mentioned that I met Dr Samiran Banerjee at Warlingham in 1949. We kept in touch and he came to work at Powick for a few months in 1953. He brought a parcel containing 6 pounds weight of the roots of the shrub *Rauwolfia serpentina benz*. I had already corresponded at length with him on the use of this root in Indian medicine. It had been known for centuries for the relief of mania, and possibly schizophrenia, but some of the indications were obscure. Like many ancient remedies its uses were diverse. There had been a revival of interest among Indian physicians and psychiatrists and a number of papers had been published. Chopra (1933) described its use in Malaya, as an anthelminthic in Java, and also for the treatment of the bites of poisonous snakes, in diarrhoea and dysentery and as an ecbolic. The way in which we set up a study to investigate its possible use in psychotherapy and psychiatry is a good indication of how one carried out research in the 1950s. The British Drug Houses ground the roots up and put them in ten-grain cachets. The dose we settled on varied from 5 to 40 grains daily. I treated 108 patients suffering from a wide variety of psychiatric conditions, and reported the results as follows (Sandison 1957):

> We have been sufficiently impressed with the clinical results obtained, to recommend the use of Rauwolfia serpentina in psychiatry as a treatment in its own right for acute and chronic psychoses and psycho-neuroses where the mental state is characterised by tension and paranoid ideas. The results appear to be permanent in a large number of cases as many of our patients were treated up to two or more years ago. It is of value in controlling tension in patients undergoing psycho-therapy, it makes life tolerable for many psycho-neurotics and it is of great value following ECT and insulin treatments. It can be used in conjunction with modified insulin treatment, alternating six weeks of each treatment, in schizophrenics in whom deep insulin treatment is contra-indicated and in anxiety neurosis. The results are least impressive in chronic psychotic patients.

Rauwolfia as a practical treatment for psychiatric illness never received much attention in the UK. For many years its synthetic derivative, rauwiloid, was used effectively for the treatment of hypertension, and I did some early trials in this field with the late Dr H.L. Milles. Supporting my twin drives towards research and 'proper doctoring', I initiated trials with thioridazine and haloperidol. This was only made possible by the appointment of Dr Eileen Whitelaw as research assistant. Rating scales were in fashion and we devised a good one, the Powick

Hospital Rating Scale (Sandison, Whitelaw and Currie 1960). The 1950s was the decade when older plant-based remedies and galenicals were replaced by laboratory generated and engineered synthetic drugs. A counter-movement to this culture was provided by the work of Michael and Enid Balint, who stressed the importance of the doctor himself in the healing equation. Their influence in general medical practice was considerable, but is largely forgotten today. Our trials with melleril and other drugs showed me that the greatly increased attention from doctors and other staff which the long-stay patients in these trials received was a significant factor in their improvement. It is a dimension hard to quantify, and thus was ignored by the editors of scientific journals. Sadly, it is easier for the psychiatrist to write a prescription for a drug, to be administered by a nurse, than to talk to the patient himself.

I have not said anything in this chapter about group work with patients at Powick, nor about the clergy group or the formation of the Worcester Samaritans. These will all appear in more appropriate places.

By 1964 I had spent 12 years working with LSD. It was exceptionally demanding work, involving participation in the patients' unconscious fantasies and experiences at an archetypal level. Some guardian angel kept me from the excesses of therapeutic enthusiasm which trapped some of my colleagues in the USA. There were those who used everything they could think of to intensify the LSD experience, as if it were not intense enough as it was. Some even took LSD with their patients, thus depriving the patient of his vital link with reality and sanity. Nevertheless, I was ready for a change. My children had grown up in a rural district of Worcestershire and learned to love its countryside. Both had left school, one to study accountancy and the other was at Cambridge. The eldest still lives in the county, while my younger son, when visiting, likes nothing better than a walk on the Malvern Hills. At the same time, my marriage had reached the point of no return. When I finally left my wife I thought we had parted in a sort of harmony. As I was getting into my car I remembered something and went back, to find her shedding bitter tears. Suddenly it was all wrong, but there was no returning. It is an image which will always be with me. Today it feels as if I had abandoned all the good I had ever meant to do. My tears were longer in coming, and when they did they were shed with an aching nostalgia for the far-off days, before the war, when a lifetime of family life and adventure seemed possible. We had travelled different pathways over the years and there was no longer a meeting point.

CHAPTER 3

In Search of a Model, 2.
SOUTHAMPTON 1964–1975

In 1964 I was appointed Consultant Psychiatrist at Knowle Hospital in Hampshire, about ten miles from Southampton. It was a difficult place to work in, very little real therapy was practised and I never saw eye to eye with the Medical Superintendent, Angus Galbraith. There were two potential bright spots in this dismal clinical scene. The Wessex School of Psychiatry had just been built in the grounds of the hospital, and another new building, the Southampton Mental Health Centre, had been located at the Royal South Hants Hospital in Southampton. The Wessex school was run by Stephen McKeith and Ian Skottowe. I got on well with both, and took part in the teaching programme, mostly on group and individual therapy. The Mental Health Centre housed all the out-patient clinics for the area, except those at Hythe and Lymington, both in the New Forest. It also contained a day hospital, which operated at the lowest possible level of clinical competence, and nobody seemed to be in charge of it.

I had given up working with LSD, and its abuse in the USA, together with its increasing street use in Britain, confirmed my view that the era was coming to an end. Although the excesses associated with LSD in the 1960s largely took place on American soil, a good deal of responsibility must rest with two British doctors, Michael Hollingshead and John Beresford. Hollingshead was described by Antonio Melechi (1997, 1998) as 'Britain's most infamous exponent of the psychedelic experience' (1997, p.87). It is a sad story, involving Timothy Leary, in which every possible cultural and moral boundary seems to have been shattered. Stories began to appear in the press of the consequences of drug abuse, including LSD, and in 1968 I was asked to act as expert adviser to the defence in the trial of Robert Lipman at the Central Criminal Court, London. He was accused of the murder of a prostitute, and his defence was that he was so under the influence of LSD that he did not know what he was doing, and that he had no recollection of harming her. It was also suggested that the girl, who had also taken LSD, might have suffocated herself. It was not a particularly savoury case. I did not give evidence, being retained to assist the defence. In the end, Lipman was acquitted of murder, and found guilty of manslaughter, and was sentenced to six years. The case was described as the first LSD murder trial in Britain, and raised some legal debating points on whether oblivion due to drugs or alcohol was a sufficient defence against a charge of murder. Lipman, in evidence, said that they both took LSD at the girl's flat, and that he went on a trip in which he plummeted into the centre of the earth and found himself in a pit full of snakes breathing fire. He thought he was in hell fighting for his life, and when he came round he found that his companion was dead beside him. The content of his fantasy was similar to that which any one of our patients could have had. In the clinical setting we would have known that it was a metaphor for the patient's psychological situation. It would have been talked through, contained and used creatively. Those, like Leary and Hollingshead, who wished to 'turn on the world' appear to have had no concept of the power of the forces they were playing with.

This was not the first time that I had appeared at the Old Bailey. During my first House job, in 1940, one of our nurses had been assaulted and raped by three Canadian soldiers. She suffered a broken jaw and other injuries, and, as I was on duty that night, I had to give evidence at the trial. It was pretty straightforward. I gave my evidence, and produced my photographs which I had taken and developed myself, and the soldiers in question went to prison for seven years. Arriving early for my case, I sat through part of the previous one, a case of unlawful wounding. The judge was summing up, and laying into an unfortunate young doctor, who had given evidence. 'He is a very junior doctor, his job was to give evidence, not opinions. He need not think he is a Bernard Spilsbury.' Sir Bernard Spilsbury was a famous and distinguished Home Office pathologist, who had a well-deserved reputation for solving some of the most difficult forensic cases of his time. It was a chance piece of advice, and which, I hope, stood me in good stead.

I have by nature and profession felt myself on the side of the underdog. I have to ask whether Robert Lipman was a villain or a victim. What purpose did six years in jail really serve? I did not suggest it, but a year in a good mental hospital might have done more for him than what the law prescribed. Indeed, during several visits to Gloucester Prison in the 1950s, I came to the conclusion that it was often a question of chance whether a man landed up in prison or in a mental hospital.

Not long after the Lipman case I was asked to appear again at the Old Bailey. It was a case which seemed to show the law at its most asinine. A warehouse had been set on fire in the East End of London and destroyed. The two men who lit the flames were in the dock. They claimed that they had been high on LSD at the time, and that claim was not disputed. One of them had been a police informer, and received a weekly sum from the police which conveniently paid for his drugs.

The police knew this and admitted it. It was an arrangement which allowed them, when it suited them, to arrest him for possession. The oddest thing of all was that the owners of the warehouse and its contents, both of which were well insured, were in considerable financial need, and they had taken the precaution of conveniently removing the contents the day before the fire. Thus it seemed to me that the real villains were never brought to justice, as I believe was the case. In evidence, I tried to argue, as had been done in the Lipman case, that the accused were so under the influence of LSD as not to be responsible for the consequences of their actions. I had not reckoned on being up against the formidable Mr Corkery, who cross-examined me for three days. Finally, I got so exasperated that I told him I had come to the court as a 'matter of conscience'. He flung down his gold pencil, repeated the word 'conscience' with some emphasis, and sat down. The judge in the case, whose name I forget, was most courteous, and after questions from him I left the box. The men were, of course, found guilty, but were sent down for only two years, reduced as they had already been in custody for six months.

During the 1960s there were many stories about disasters while under the effects of LSD. Some, like the teenager who jumped off the roof of a chapel because he thought he could fly, and the Californians who were blinded because they believed they could outstare the sun, were later shown to be false. Others were well founded. Nevertheless, when one considers the many millions of people who took LSD in unsuitable and unsupervised environments, the number of casualties and criminal acts was probably surprisingly low. In the field of therapy, Stanislav Grof (1975) reported that most of the criticisms of LSD therapy had been directed at methodology, and that 'no-one had questioned the safety of this approach' (p.2).

The Southampton years marked the end of my association with mental hospitals. My frustration with the increasing dependence on the prescription of psychotropic drugs which characterised the work of most of my colleagues emerged in a paper (R. Sandison 1972). This paper also records the increasing lack of communication and understanding between doctors and administrators, and the way in which patients were being controlled in increasingly subtle ways.

About 1968 I was approached by the staff of the extramural department of Southampton University with a view to taking part in the development of group work courses. I joined the Group Analytic Society (London) about this time. The plan was for a three-day workshop for three groups, each led by two facilitators. The first of these workshops was held in September 1969 and staffed by four members from the academic department of social work, the psychologist Cary Cooper, and myself. The workshop attracted 30 participants, and was followed by 30 weekly meetings. The latter were not a great success after the intensity of the workshop, and were reduced in number and altered in character subsequently.

After the first year we asked Peter Smith, a sociologist and group analyst from Sussex University, to act as our consultant. I was associated with this annual workshop until 1975, and over the years we made continual changes which improved the quality of the work.

This group brought home to me the importance of the setting. We met successively in the Department of Sociology, the Maths Building of the University, and finally at the Wickham Pastoral Centre, situated at a convent about ten miles from Southampton. The sociology department had too many work associations with most of the staff members, the maths building was a concrete jungle and a near disaster, while the pastoral centre seemed perfectly in tune with our ethos. The religious setting was there, but not intrusive, and everyone agreed that whether they were 'believers' or not, it was as near perfect a setting as possible. There is a religious dimension to all small groups, and many large groups.

All this took place during the time that I was trying to rebuild and make sense of my life after the break with Evelyn. It was far more difficult than I had anticipated. I recall that my father had died in 1959. I agree with the view that the death of the father is the most important psychological event in a man's life. It gave me the freedom to start the process which I thought would free me from a claustrophobic marriage. I remarried in 1965. We had many clinical interests in common, but our social and cultural backgrounds could scarcely have been more different. I was drawn by an unconscious force which persuaded me that, LSD not being any longer available, I could, like Simon of my novel, experience 'the greatest love affair in the world'. When Jung was engaged in talking to his anima, and she told him that he was the greatest psychologist in the world, he commented, 'Then I knew she was lying!' Unfortunately, and significantly, I recorded no dreams between the late 1950s and 1975, which indicates my state of unconsciousness during those years. You could say that I was deceived by my anima.

My compensatory mechanisms were not limited to constructing and rebuilding in the clinical field, I launched into the rebuilding of houses. However, I was not able to enjoy the results; as soon as they were finished I had to move. The result was two pleasant homes in Hampshire, for someone else. I did not stop there. Something was drawing me back to Shetland, and I bought a derelict croft house at Clousta in 1968, which I restored over the next few years. I was evidently still searching for my great love. The great mother comes to mind.

Something parallel was happening in my professional life. I left the security of mental hospital life, and I suppose that was a kind of divorce. I had worked in that environment for over twenty years. There were plenty of derelict psychological buildings in Southampton, and a lot of opportunity to erect new structures. I spent a couple of years transforming the day hospital from a dismal occupation centre into a therapeutic community. It was an immensely rewarding project, and I believe it was a happy place to work in, and that we did some good to the patients.

I have always believed that the key people in a successful psychiatric unit are the consultant and the ward sister or charge nurse. This combination, if successful, works like a good marriage. Good marriages beget healthy children in various forms, and, at the day hospital, I regarded the staff sensitivity group as a family meeting. Most of the therapy with the patients was in groups, and among these was the group for psychotic patients which I wrote up at a later date (Sandison 1991, 1994).

Inevitably, schizophrenic patients in varying stages of remission were referred to the day hospital. They were not easy to integrate into the group activities, and I decided to establish a special therapy group for them. There were ten patients and four staff members, and the group met for 40 minutes five days a week. There are a good many reports in the literature of group work with schizophrenics, but I do not know of any where so many staff were involved. The staff were myself, a registrar, a senior nurse and a student nurse. After each meeting the staff met for 30 minutes, one of whom wrote up each day's events. Not all the patients attended every day. Some came late, some walked out. An average attendance was seven members. We felt we could tolerate this behaviour in view of the otherwise strong boundary structure of the group. The latter created a sense of authority and sanity.

The group met for five months, and I feel that most of the patients benefited. It was also a valuable learning experience for the staff. Some of its success can be attributed to the fact that it took place within the setting of the daily community meeting, or 'holding group', which contained many of the tensions and chaotic feelings which stalked through the day hospital. Within these boundaries patients felt much more free to express strong feelings, including their psychotic fantasies and experiences. In line with my belief that sanity and insanity lie on the same continuum, it seemed appropriate that the staff should, when the moment seemed right, share their own experiences with the group.

At first, issues of trust were more pressing than in most therapy groups. The psychotic is careful with whom he shares his inner fantasies.

> One day a patient spoke of his bizarre experiences of metamorphosis; for example, how, in hospital, the nurse would turn into the devil, or into a bird. He was asked why he hadn't talked about this before. He replied, 'Some of you might have found it upsetting; I didn't want to upset anyone.' A sense of human feeling and detachment was evident. On another occasion a patient talked about a patient he knew, not a member of the group, who believed he could walk across the River Thames without sinking: 'Of course I knew it was nonsense,' he said, 'and I told him so!'

On another occasion visual hallucinations were being discussed:

> A patient turned to me and said rather aggressively, 'How can you understand this, you've never been hallucinated?' Without going into detail, I told him of two occasions on which I had seen a vision. He didn't ask the details, it was

enough that he knew that I had a personal understanding of his inner world. On another occasion a patient told the group about a very traumatic abortion she had had which had triggered her psychosis. Rather to my surprise, the student nurse then described her own abortion experience, again without going into detail. It was enough to create the longed-for bridge between sanity and insanity. It helped that great universal cry to be met, the need to be understood and heard.

Following the same star we introduced some simple 'trust' exercises:

The staff were Ronnie, David and Barbara and the patients were Raymond, Patrick, Hazel, Wendy, Derek, Helen and Angela. The group stood up and linked hands. Patrick had been lying on the floor 'because of his back' but he got up and joined in with no sign of pain. He then said that he had never been able to trust therapy, but he could trust people. He felt a lot of power running through the group. He felt that everyone was a battery. (One of his psychotic ideas was that he needed to be 'charged up' and sometimes he would run the engine of his car and grasp the spark plugs to receive this charge.) Raymond felt very uneasy and said that he had shaken hands with a lot of people but they had all let him down. He told David that he thought the doctors were praying for magical healing powers. Barbara asked if he would feel safer in the centre of the group. When there he seemed easier, but said that he felt like a wet frog. Later I asked the group if they felt any closer to each other. Wendy, Derek and Helen said immediately that they heard voices. The next day Wendy suggested that the group should hold hands. They did this but showed more anxiety than hitherto. Derek asked for an explanation of what we were doing and for references to the literature which would support it. Raymond said that it was all right as they had done it as kids. In earlier sessions several patients had talked about being cut off from childhood and of having lost their sense of fun (loss of wit = lost wits = madness). Now they could return to childhood and they discovered that it was an anxious process. There may also have been references to childhood sexuality and to sexual anxiety. Their ambivalence was revealed by the fact that on that day the patients did not want to leave when time was up. The following day was a point of climax for the group. When time was up, Hazel, who had hitherto said nothing, said that she did not want to leave and started talking about her mother in a very angry and paranoid fashion, adding that she always had to be nice to her and that it was only 'down here' that she could let herself go. Eventually I said that it was long after time and that the group must end, whereupon she became very angry with me saying that whenever she wanted to talk to me I always had something else to do. She then became quite out of control, attacking me with her fists and saying she wanted to kill me. By this time all the group had left except Robin (a patient) and Barbara. Eventually I managed to hold her and told her that she really wanted to kill someone else. She shouted: 'You know who it is!' I said: 'Yes, but you have to say it.' She then shouted: 'It's my bloody mother!' The next day we asked Hazel to go into the centre of the group and fight her way out. She did this, whereupon Helen exclaimed: 'We've hit Aquarius!'

How are we to understand this episode? The group itself had been Hazel's ego boundary which she could not leave for fear that she would once more fall into the hands of mother. The conflict was forced on her by my saying that the group must end. The psychotic part of her might interpret this as saying that the group had ended for ever. She saw me nevertheless as one capable of enabling her to join the opposites. Thus she was faced with the choice of killing me or her mother. Still unresolved, the group recognised intuitively that Hazel must experience the strength of the ego as represented by breaking out of the encircling group. At this point Helen said 'We've hit Aquarius!', or, one might say, the opposites had been reconciled.

This may be an appropriate point at which to comment on the way in which the patients linked the concept of 'closeness' with the hearing of voices. I understand this as meaning that something had happened to each of them, which allowed them to link their feelings at a single level. In the group I came to understand that each patient's fantasy world (projected as 'hallucinations') was personal and not necessarily understood or even recognised by another psychotic. It was as if an engineer started talking with a scholar of ancient Greek and a third person assumed that they were talking about the same thing. In this case, the individual psychotic patient's experience is not only unique but essential to his or her fragile integrity. To say that the experience could cross personal boundaries was taking a considerable risk. This was demonstrated by the fact that on the following day, when the group joined hands, they all showed much more anxiety. There is one other matter, which is hard to fit into any attempt to analyse the occurrence in that group. Throughout the life of the group, although many bizarre things happened, there seemed a sort of rightness or sanity about them at the time, as if they belonged to the natural order of things. Fifteen years later it feels different, but I still instinctively hesitate to dissect it too far.

What happened to these people? Six months later we did a follow-up. Raymond was still attending the day hospital and being considered for a new group. Patrick was also still at the day hospital and was reported to be 'moving nearer to a job'. Hazel was working but had had one hospital admission since the group ended. Wendy was working as a nursing assistant with a view to nursing training. Derek was 'working'. Helen was at art college and looking after her children again. Angela was working, which we thought was quite an achievement, as she had previously had four hospital admissions in two years.

This extract from the life of the group can only provide a taste of what happened. One of the functions of the group was to give orderliness and coherence to the jangle of sounds varying from extreme regression to adult concern, from psychosis and fantasy to sanity and reality. The group could never be the whole treatment; it was part of an integral programme.

In the 1994 paper I sought to extend my understanding of the schizophrenic process. This quest has been a recurring theme during my professional life, and there are still many unanswered questions. What 'fixes' a delusional idea or system and renders it impermeable to reason or the evidence of reality? What sudden eruption of the unconscious links a stranger's face with the patient's belief that his wife is being unfaithful? In the following extracts I followed the fortunes of Helen, whose name has been mentioned as a member of the group when Hazel went out of control. This account starts when the group was young, having just completed its third session.

> After the third group session David (staff) said that he was amazed at the depths to which patients might go. He recalled that Helen had talked about her childhood, which to him was all new. She had talked about her father trying to knife her mother when she was a child. Helen said this in response to another patient who said he had a strong feeling that he would knife someone one day.

From the beginning, two patterns frequently appeared: first, that a fantasy or psychotic statement uttered by one patient would evoke remembered material from another; second, all the patients reported chaotic and schismatic families, in which parental strife, violence and separation were common. As it became safe to explore personal psychotic themes, preoccupation with sex, death and violence, which were often interchangeable, became powerfully evident.

A dream early in psychotherapy may set the tone for the whole analysis. Similarly, the early happenings in the group deserve special notice.

> On that third day Helen said that she was trying to say a lot, but couldn't make herself understood, so she was blocked. A staff member noticed that Helen said that everyone coughed when she wanted to speak, but that it was Helen herself who had a coughing fit and had to go out. Thus Helen's contribution to the first layer, so to say, of the matrix was to project her fantasy on to all the other group members. Owing to the relative parity in numbers between staff and patients the patients were quick to notice that their roles were different. They agreed that the patients had something wrong with them, but what about the staff? David (staff) drew the group's attention to the fact that no one knew whether the staff had anything wrong with them or not. Later in the life of the group there were references to the staff of mental hospitals being 'as nutty as the patients', while the group made some great leaps forward when the time came for the staff to declare their own humanity and their own 'other selves' as able to resonate with psychotic experience. Early attempts to achieve this were an important attempt on the part of the whole group to close the circle of the matrix and to give it a more uniform psychotic content. The very next day there was confirmation of this when Helen had to leave the group after talking about her paranoid feelings.

After she left, the discussion about this was interrupted by Hazel (patient) asking David (staff) why he was wearing a pink shirt. It was her attempt to point out that each member of the group, staff and patients alike, had some unique quirk.

When it seemed to me that there was some group cohesion I suggested some simple 'trust exercises', which usually involved standing or sitting in a circle and holding hands. I described some aspects of the effect this had on the group in the 1991 paper. Developing this now, it was noticed that the group began to express sexual anxieties and some of the group identified the holding of hands with sexual intercourse. One woman said she was about to explode but realised that it would 'soon be over'.

Helen remarked that she hadn't been home to her parents at the weekend.

Once the sexual theme had been liberated it gained strength. Helen spoke of her father's attempted seduction of her when she was 16 and of her abortion at the age of 22, and that she had told no one including her parents and her therapist. It was then that Sue (staff) said that she had had the same experience, which Helen said helped her a lot. These reality experiences gave permission for other patients to examine their sexual fantasies. Raymond (patient) said that his ambition was to be locked in a room with 20 women who would all attack him in turn. Someone asked if he wanted them to be nude.

From sex we moved to violence. Helen described her aversion to meat, linking this to her father's experiences with the Mau Mau in Kenya and her mother's suicidal bid. Not eating meat was her way of denying nourishment to her aggressive self.

As the group developed these themes there was a mass of material about parental discord, double binds, breakdown of parents' marriages and the sense of loss created by all this. It gave credence to Fromm-Reichmann's concept of the schizophrenogenic mother (1959), to Bateson et al.'s (1956) double bind and to Lidz's (1975) concepts of schismatic and skewed family types. The latter formulates schizophrenia as 'a failure to differentiate properly between the self and others and between what arises within the self and what is outside the self'.

There were other themes which helped to complete the picture of the culture and matrix of this group. There was a constant shuttling between inner and outer, which I understand as an important part of the healing process. For example, after Helen's metaphorical statement 'We've hit Aquarius!', Robin (patient) was repeatedly questioned about why he laughed so much. His reply was to talk about the Isle of Wight. Attempts by the group to rationalise psychotic behaviour often followed this pattern.

Psychotic secrets were being revealed all the time, as we have seen. Sexual secrets accompanied them, but had more to do with reality than fantasy. As the group developed it spent more time talking about the realities of life, about leaving the day hospital, getting a job, resuming social relationships. There was always a respect for the psychotic ideas and experiences of others, and a belief that each person possessed something unique and valuable. I have barely mentioned the themes of evolution, of reincarnation and of understanding of the cosmos which were woven into the group matrix. Helen wished to know why she was here. She felt frustrated because she could not remember the past lives she believed she had lived. Patrick (patient) also believed in reincarnation, and had been to the library to ask for the 56 volumes on Germany which he believed he had written in a previous life. Hence this theme was about the two selves, the irrational buried self and the rational self. Helen once said: 'Wouldn't it be funny if we all began as an amoeba and progressed up through rats etc. to human beings?' I felt that this was a metaphor for the development of the group and that she was preparing herself to leave. She did this when she got a place in art college, and six months later she was doing well and able to resume the care of her two children.

This work at the day hospital was succeeded by the opening of the Southampton Psychotherapy Department in 1973, which was requested by the Wessex Regional Board, and warmly supported by my colleagues. An account of how this came about and the process by which it was achieved was published in *Group Analysis* (Sandison and Sevitt 1977). The following is adapted from the first part.

Part 1 – The formation of the Department of Psychotherapy

A number of considerations led me to believe, several years ago, that it should be possible to provide adequate psychotherapy for NHS patients. First of all I started to think about the qualities needed by a psychotherapist, and it seemed that they were such that with adequate training and supervision they could be fostered and developed in a wide variety of professional people. I had in mind nurses, social workers, teachers and others. The discipline of training, self-knowledge and the experience of people thus gained are important. Also necessary are personal qualities such as warmth, the ability for self-criticism, openness to personal change, willingness to take risks, to be challenging, the patience to see therapy through and the personal integrity and discipline to set up and maintain a healthy therapeutic contract with the patient. It became the task of the medical psychotherapist in the Department to recognise these potential qualities and to provide opportunities for their growth and development.

Other considerations which led to the formation of the Department were my own dissatisfactions about what happens in most psychiatric Out Patients' Departments. Psychiatrists in Out Patients are often caught between pressures from the patients and the general practitioner on the one hand and their own desire to render a service on the other. The result is often a collusive interaction leading to short interviews with a large number of patients at relatively long intervals. Patient dependency prevents them from moving out of the sick role… It has often occurred to me as odd that in-patients receive most of their therapy from nurses, since the doctors have several wards and far too many patients to treat, whilst out-patients receive all their treatment from doctors. There has been a resistance to putting out-patient nurses in a therapeutic role.

I had been addressing the question of how this group of professional people could be trained to become therapists in the NHS. for some years. The beginnings of an answer came in Southampton in 1967 when I was approached by some university staff and asked to take part in a training course in group dynamics for social workers. This led to the first one week intensive group work course run by the University of Southampton Extra-mural Department. Fortunately, it was realised at the start that the course would be enriched by being multi-disciplinary and on that first course in 1968 some NHS. staff, including nurses, attended. Briefly, it was a one week intensive sensitivity course followed by a series of weekly groups. Some participants took part in an advanced course, which included theoretical training. These University courses ran successfully for several years and have now been superseded by similar courses run by the Department of Psychotherapy. Various members of hospital staff who attended the first course had a difficult time when they returned to their everyday work, as their new-found skills and personal growth were often treated with scepticism and anxiety by colleagues. Gradually, however, as the numbers of people who had been on the course increased there came a point of no return. There was a strong movement in the area to offer patients psychotherapy whenever appropriate, and to use psycho-dynamic skills to work more effectively in multi-disciplinary teams and to communicate more openly with colleagues. It was at this point that organisation became essential.

The organisation of psychotherapy in Southampton came about simultaneously in several areas. Personally, I had been devoting my energies to treating a therapeutic community in the Day Hospital, using this as a training ground for nurses, social workers and occupational therapists in group and individual therapy. At the same time a group of about 12 people had been meeting at my house every month to discuss various aspects of psychotherapy. A supervision seminar in psychotherapy was started for registrars, whilst more time was made available in the Diploma of Psychological Medicine (DPM) course for teaching this subject. Individuals in other areas were starting groups of their own, both inside and outside the hospital.

The three organisational principles which make for a successful programme in psychotherapy are as follows:

1. There must be skilled assessment of the patient's suitability for psychotherapy and of the appropriate type of therapy in which to place him or her.

2. There must be provision for attracting, training and supervising a numerically adequate body of therapists.

3. There must be an umbrella psychotherapy department which co-ordinates the various psychotherapeutic activities and thus ensures that there is a proper balance of therapies available.

The Department of Psychotherapy at the Royal South Hants Hospital was formed using these principles. It took place on the eve of a cool financial climate and material resources were severely limited. I realised that my role would be one of organisation and training and that my skills as a psychotherapist would be largely devoted to selecting and training potential therapists. The core of the Department was tiny and even after two years there were only three of us whose major commitment was to the Department. I had a part-time (6 sessions a week) contract as Consultant Psychotherapist, and there was a full time secretary and a full time nurse therapist. There were also a few people who had some 'official' sessions in the Department but whose principle job was elsewhere. There was another group of people who gave regular time to psychotherapy but who had no official sessions with the team. Beyond these again was a fairly large group of about 20 or more who were involved as co-therapists in groups, in conjoint marital therapy and in some individual therapy. These were drawn from many disciplines, and many were from outside the National Health Service. Within the NHS nurses were well represented. Outside it there were staff from the University Department of Sociology, from Social Services, the Church and Teaching. When people came from outside the Health Service our only stipulation was that they should work with or under the supervision of an NHS person.

In part 2, we examined what happened to the 172 patients who were referred to the department during the first 15 months of its operation. I left the department at the end of 1975, when Dr Pamela Ashurst succeeded me as consultant psychotherapist. As far as I am aware it continues to flourish today, despite very large changes in the organisation of psychiatry in Southampton during the past 25 years. The 'holding group' for the heterogeneous collection of therapists working in the department was the Wessex Psychotherapy Society. The Society ran an annual three-day conference and workshop at the newly opened medical school from 1973 onwards which was attended by about 150 people. I believe that gives a true indication of the desire locally to have and to take part in a psychiatric service whose orientation was psychotherapeutic.

The Medical School at Southampton was being planned and developed during most of my time in the area, and accepted its first students in 1972. I particularly welcomed the introduction of the students to patients and their families in the first year, and the elective fourth year studies. Some came to the department of psychotherapy where they were not only welcomed, but contributed usefully to the work. The Committee on Medical Education, chaired by Lord Todd, had reported in 1968, and its recommendations had far-reaching results, particularly in post-graduate education. General practitioners were expected to work in the psychiatric field as part of their training. All these developments were new and exciting, and I extended my teaching programme accordingly.

I was particularly glad when I was invited to join the selection committee for medical students. In its first year after opening, the University accepted 80 students, rising to 120 during the next two years. There were 1200 applicants each year, and selection was therefore a formidable task. Unfortunately, and probably inevitably, selection was largely by school reports and by projections about 'A' level results. Only about ten candidates each year were interviewed. Some of these came to me because of some doubt about their psychiatric history. I do not recall any who were turned down on this account. Although the educational requirements were rigid, two 'A's and a 'B' at 'A' level, there was some flexibility. We tried to give preference to local candidates and those whose first preference was Southampton; we had a small quota for overseas students, and we took a few mature, post-graduate students each year. The requirements excluded many. Those with a classical education were very few, and I always felt particular sadness when a young man or woman from a medical family failed to make it on educational grounds. So often they were among the most strongly motivated candidates. No doubt selection procedures have changed and moved on since 1975. This medical school opened at a time when the National Health Service was riding high, and large numbers of able and strongly motivated young men and women were keen to take part. Things may be different today.

The internal forces which resulted in my leaving this interesting life and thriving medical scene are not clear to me even today. In the spring of 1975 I went to a conference in Glasgow, where I met Malcolm Millar, professor of psychiatry in Aberdeen. I discussed my developing thoughts about moving to Shetland, and he suggested that I might like to combine it with some teaching work for the diploma course in psychotherapy, for which Aberdeen was the pioneer. This not only excited my interest in going north, but it satisfied some of my need for recognition which has dogged me for most of my life.

I left Southampton in November 1975, amid many expressions of goodwill from my colleagues and friends. I think there was a general expectation that I was going to Shetland to retire and lead a country life in the land of my fathers. I was following whatever fate had for me. My second marriage had merely increased the number of my dependants, but it gave me no fire. I still had to rely on my inner need to find a derelict house, or hospital, or person, or some barren psychological soil, to nurture and build afresh, and then hope that it could manage by itself. The institutions I had given life to in Southampton were in good hands, and they did survive. It was my own psychological survival which I came to question more and more over the next few years.

CHAPTER 4

In Search of a Model, 3. SHETLAND and ABERDEEN 1975–1982

The forces which impelled me to spend these seven years in Shetland were indeed deep and complex. Among their components was a desire to live out the kind of life experienced by my ancestors, which I had been denied. Uncle Jack, whose stories about medical practice there had once been my model for the ideal doctor, had died before I qualified. I saw myself as carrying a torch for him once more in the place he had known and loved. On my summer visits I had heard about and been saddened by the primitive way that psychiatric patients were treated, and I was fired to do something to change this. There had never been a resident psychiatrist in Shetland, despite population figures which would have fully justified such an appointment. Every two months two psychiatrists from Aberdeen spent about two weeks in Shetland. Between these visits, any psychiatric patient requiring more than the general practitioners could offer was sent to Aberdeen, 200 miles south of Lerwick, by sea or air. The cost of this was formidable, and would have paid the salaries of a consultant and some supporting staff with ease. The Shetland Health Board was highly conservative and did not agree.

I always felt at a disadvantage. I had lived and worked almost all my life in England. I had lost my Shetland accent. The only thing that gave me a Shetland identity was the spelling of my name, and among those who knew me, recollections of my family. I would probably have fared better in Lerwick, the capital, but a curious fate drew me to the north of the mainland, where my ancestors had once lived. In 1974 I bought the derelict Haa of Ollaberry, not knowing at the time that it had strong associations with my great-great-grandfather, whose biography I was to write years later. The Haa houses of Shetland were mostly built in the 17th and 18th centuries and were the seats of the lairds, or landowners. They were all of Scots origin and were generally disliked, if not hated, despite the fact that many were caring and generous to their tenants. Their reputation as greedy incomers persists to this day. The Haa houses of Shetland were not large, but when they were built they were big compared with the small dwellings occupied by most Shetland families. The Haa of Ollaberry had a peculiar appeal to me. The walls and the stairwell were sound, most of the rest had to be rebuilt. It lay on the shore with its own pier, beach, three derelict cottages, and a deserted wool mill. All of these were restored in time except for the mill. The latter had been used as a place of worship for many years during the 19th century until the present church was opened in 1867, the old Kirk being ruined. I was unaware of this also at the time.

I cannot speak too highly of the devotion and generosity with which the local men set about the work of restoration. The oil industry was building the giant oil terminal at Sullom Voe a few miles away, which would transform and change the island economy and way of life of many people for ever. Large numbers of incomers returned, some of them Shetlanders in exile, like myself. The fervour with which Tommy Mouat and his team went about their work was, I believe, to do with their own need to preserve, restore and hold on to their traditions.

In the month in which I moved to Shetland I had a dream. It followed an earlier dream in which I meet my analyst who asks me why I am always dreaming about France, to which I reply that I never dreamt about it. But later that night I dreamt that I was in the Loire Valley, making a circular tour of discovery, and in the succeeding months I had repeated dreams of that country. The dream during my removal was about a great inter-continental train which steams up from France en route for Aberdeen. My wife was at the controls and the train was derailed. We cannot get the locomotive back on its track without massive help, cranes, platelayers, mechanics.

The dream must speak for itself. My wife never saw anything wrong with the marriage, I knew that it had become derailed long before, and that it was beyond me to restore it, even if I had wished to. The question was: when should it be buried? In another dream shortly after the last I am in my personal house, in the 'bedchamber'. They bring in a dead Frenchman. There is a ritual to be observed at his burial using a black quilt. But the dead man has to say when he is ready to be buried. I am an artist and fear the loss of my paints. The Frenchman draws my attention to some earth pigments in a pot and tells me that they are inexhaustible and that they will always be there. Then he says that he is ready to be buried.

Clearly the Frenchman had to be listened to. I knew I was in Shetland with the wrong person. I had known the person I longed for since 1969. The derailing process had begun even before that date. Certain developments had to occur before the burial could take place, and it was not until 1982 that Beth and I were able to be together.

Creating a psychodynamic climate in Shetland was exactly like setting out to make a painting by digging the pigments out of the earth and refining them oneself. By working more closely with the social work department than with the doctors I gradually established a base at the health centre in Lerwick. The general practitioners were generally suspicious of specialists. They felt that they were, in a remote island group, emotionally and intellectually equipped to deal with any medical situation. The first consultant surgeon was Rose-Innes, appointed in 1923, and between 1975 and 1982 the surgeon was still single handed. I met a need, but it was accepted reluctantly and with much ambivalence. One practitioner, who was a good friend, told me one day that he had no need of a psychiatrist, he could handle all his patients himself. The very next day he referred a depressed patient to me, but he never saw any incongruity in this action. Similarly, a Lerwick doctor strongly vetoed my request that a bed in the hospital should be designated as a mental health bed under the Act. His grounds were that the nurses could not handle such cases, which was nonsense. The very next day he, without batting an eyelid, asked me to see a disturbed patient who he had admitted to the hospital. Over the years he probably referred more patients to me than anyone else, and we had an excellent professional and personal rapport. I chaired the medical committee for six years, I believe with success. I think the GPs liked this as it kept out the consultant surgeon, who had some ideas they did not favour. There were many small power struggles, but in an island community, as in a large family, the status quo has to be maintained at all costs.

Professionally it could have been a lonely life, had it not been for my monthly visit to Aberdeen. The diploma course in psychotherapy had almost collapsed two years previously, due to the unacceptable behaviour of one of the members of the teaching staff. It had been a painful and damaging episode and nobody wished to talk about it. This seemed healthy as there was a massive urge to regenerate the course, and much excitement and enthusiasm at the prospect. Malcolm Millar, who had been analysed by Fairbairn, was probably the only professor of psychiatry at the time who could claim to be an analyst. The course was run on a group dynamics basis, and my task was to do some teaching on Jung and to act as consultant to the staff group. The whole group was full of energy and worked immensely hard, discussion and planning going on till late evening. It was an atmosphere which I enjoyed, thrived on and learnt much from.

My lecture, or, rather, seminar, contributions to the course were more of a collection of topics which were around at the time rather than a course based on a theme. I seldom lectured 'on Jung', preferring to give a Jungian flavour to my material wherever appropriate. I still keep those files full of notes, but they read differently today. At the time they were vibrant and full of life, resonating as they were with the needs and issues of the moment. Group work developed, and it was not long before we were running three-day group work courses on the

Southampton model. These culminated in a combined exercise with the Group Analytic Society (London), who arranged for four members of the society to come north to help us run a regional group dynamics course at Edzell Grange. Despite some extraordinary fantasies in the society's committee about the state of psychoanalysis in Scotland this was a great success. It was probably the first time that the society realised that group analysis was alive and well outside London and that it could help nurture it.

To continue would be to offer a rather monotonous catalogue. I had a very enjoyable, rewarding and exciting few years in Aberdeen. This started to draw to a close when Douglas Haldane was appointed as full-time senior lecturer in 1979, and Bill Brough as consultant psychotherapist. I was consulted about the latter appointment and strongly advised the medical committee not to appoint a psychotherapist without the expectation that he would head a department of psychotherapy. Professor Millar had retired. Had he been there I think this is what would have happened, but my proposal was ignored and Bill had a very unhappy three years before leaving to return to England. Meanwhile I transferred my energies to the day hospital, run by Ken Morrice. Ken and I had much in common, and he was a poet. When I left the Aberdeen scene in 1982 it had been much transformed. The process of transformation I had witnessed and taken some part in. I recall now that metamorphosis had formed the title of one of my early lectures. Quoting from Ovid's *Metamorphosis*, I observed that the process of transformation classically resulted in many adventures involving pain, humiliation and suffering, but in the end enrichment of life. I was no doubt thinking of Lucius transformed into an ass by mistake when he had wished to be a bird. I also remember that it was his lover who brought him the wrong ointment which started his apparent misfortunes in the first place. I observed in my lecture that men are changed by others, whereas women change themselves. In the latter case I was thinking of Pallas Athene, whose life and magical powers much exercised me at that time.

At the beginning of 1977 I received a phone call from the Kensington and Chelsea Health Authority. I had been in Shetland for a little over a year. A new roof covered the Haa of Ollaberry. Much remained to be done and we were living in one of the cottages. The caller asked if I would join an enquiry tribunal in London as its medical member. The enquiry was about some unhappy goings-on at the Paddington Day Hospital and would take about three weeks. Always keen for a diversion and for a new experience, and reassured by the time estimate, I accepted. I should not have been so naïve, the enquiry lasted most of that year, cost a vast sum of money and we finally wrote the report in January 1978. It resulted in the dismissal of a consultant, but the process destroyed the day hospital and almost wrecked its parent, the Paddington Centre for Psychotherapy, hitherto one of the bright spots in the health service and a centre of excellence.

The enquiry was held in the Great Western Hotel, one of the Great Western Railway's flagships in the days of steam. I lived there throughout, except for a break in August. The legal process demonstrated the use of the adversarial system at its worst. It was like using the proverbial sledgehammer to crack a nut, only the nut kept rolling away into a corner and it usually took several days to find, only for the same process to be repeated. The health authority were extra-ordinarily generous to me over expenses, travel and entertainment, but I reflected that every time I indulged myself was a loss to patients. One could either abandon oneself to the madness of the whole enterprise and take advantage of the system, or adopt a kind of puritanical innocence. The latter was not exactly in my nature, and I adopted a middle course, taking the enquiry very seriously, and nurturing myself as required the rest of the time.

Beth moved to London not long after I left Southampton, where she continued teaching special needs children. Her presence there was clearly part of the equation and we met regularly. Fate had played a hand again. I learned that it was Irvine Kreeger, consultant psychotherapist at King's, who had suggested my name for the enquiry. He had been a good friend and had given me much good advice and practical help when I was setting up the department of psychotherapy in Southampton. I think he was much loved at King's and told me once that the staff knew him there as 'sex and death Kreeger', as these were two subjects he used to lecture to nurses. He was a keen observer and when he lectured once in Southampton he spent most of his talk analysing the occasion when he was 20 minutes late for his afternoon session. It was a talk that was spellbinding. Sadly, he died painfully a few years later. Beth and I feel that he was part of the fate that determined our future. It was as if we had been washed up on the same beach together and needed to recognise the apparent coincidence. Those who are ship-wrecked move slowly, and we were no exception.

On 8 November at about 5pm, I was discussing the day's proceedings with Hazel Counsel, the chairman of the tribunal, when the telephone rang. My elder son told me that Evelyn had been involved in a very serious car accident that morning, that she was in hospital, and that she might not live. He and my younger son Johnnie were at the hospital and they thought it better if I stayed in London. Beth came over that evening, and at about 9 in the evening Chris rang again to say that she had died. At that moment the years rolled away and it was as if we had been together, just as close as we once were, until that last day when she set off with her sister to drive to London. On that day the years of strife, the separation, the divorce and the resulting silence no longer existed. Apart from Beth, I have never expected anyone else to understand this. She and her sister are buried with their parents in the churchyard of St Mary's, Felpham, in West Sussex. It is a beautiful Norman church where we were married more than 38 years earlier, and the village is a place we had known and loved since childhood. We never consciously met there as children, but it was a strange conjunction of places and events which brought us together. Felpham is a place of pilgrimage for me to this day, and both my parents lie in the same churchyard. Life is full of contradictions. Evelyn's parents, who lived separate lives from the time she was born, lie in the same grave. My parents, who were never physically far apart, are buried in separate parts of the churchyard. It was my mother's wish.

The enquiry pursued its remorseless progress. Evelyn, by her death, had more influence on my life than ever before. She had bitter feelings towards my second wife. Once she mentioned one or two names of people she would have been happy for me to marry. I like to think that Beth would have been one of them. However, I felt a freedom to make some decisions about my future, but agonised greatly over what they should be. It took me a long time to let Evelyn go. Three years later I dreamt that she was waking up after the accident, and that her injuries were quite slight. But I could not see her face.

Returning to Shetland I went to see my old friend Albert Hunter, one of the few Shetlanders of his generation to return to Shetland after medical school to practice there. By a strange coincidence his wife had been killed in a road accident the day after Evelyn died. It was a uniquely bonding conjunction, and we did much mourning together. Thus it was that I carried my grief back to the land of my fathers and buried it there, or some of it.

What I was trying to do professionally began to take shape. There were 17 inhabited islands in the group, of which Mainland is the largest. I could seldom get to the less accessible ones and never went to Fair Isle. I planned to visit once a month those on which there was a doctor, and these visits were welcomed and useful. In doing this I was clearly living out my uncle's stories of his journeys and the romance was still there. I visited many patients in their homes. It was always a puzzle and an ethical dilemma when asked to see a psychotic patient living alone in a rather remote croft who was creating anxiety among the neighbours. People could tolerate eccentricity, but psychosis alarmed them. I recall an elderly lady who farmed her own land. I started off badly. The gate to her land had a large gap in the fence on one side. Rather than open the gate I walked through the gap. Observing this my patient decided that I was another one of her persecutors. I solved this awkwardness by retracing my steps and coming in again through the gate, which apparently satisfied her. The social workers wanted her removed to Kingseat Hospital in Aberdeen. I was on the patient's side, and fought for her to stay. I had also to pacify her neighbours who were alarmed by her psychotic behaviour, in which she often shouted obscenities and threatened to kill people. Another patient was also living alone in her croft house. In the porch was a large piece of skate. The smell of fish was strong, but nothing to the atmosphere inside, where I met my patient surrounded by the 35 cats she kept. The skate had come from the local fishermen, who dropped off any unwanted fish as they passed. She too was psychotic, but I managed to keep her at home, and she eventually got together with a man who was almost equally mentally unstable but it seemed to work.

I found myself up against authority again when I was asked to see a girl of 13 who refused to go to school. She was apparently perfectly happy working round the croft, and saw no reason to go to Lerwick and live in a hostel and sit in a classroom. I could not help being on her side, but the law said differently. Inevitably I lost the battle and she was taken to Lerwick, where I later learned that she had 'settled down well'. I wondered exactly what that meant, but I was not asked to see her again.

I held my clinics in Lerwick and they were always rewarding. I had some resonance with Carl Meier's statement years before, that the uneducated peasants were the patients who understood unconscious process better than any other. The people of Shetland would be rightly offended by being called peasants, and education has always been valued and sought after, but most live far closer to the earth and nature in its manifold varieties than any other group I have worked with. I recall a patient who lived on a remote croft. She was aged about 70, a widow of over 30 years. She lived alone, although close to her daughter and grand-daughter, and she had developed an irrational fear of dogs, an awkward problem in sheep country. The dog which gave her the greatest anxiety, however, belonged to her grand-daughter, a pretty and sexually liberated young woman. In trying to help this patient I found myself hampered by the sexual taboo. She was elderly and appeared quite unworldly. She came to my aid one day when she said, 'I wonder, doctor, if it is all due to sex?' It was this remark that liberated me, and I immediately understood the symbolism of the dog belonging to her sexually active grand-daughter, and its effect in awaking long-dormant sexual desires.

Shetlanders took readily to the concept of family therapy. In the South there is usually resistance, the patient and his or her relatives insisting that they are the problem, and that it is nothing to do with the others. There it was different; my suggestion that I, and usually a social worker, could come to their home seemed to most a very natural way of dealing with the problem. I think the Shetlanders are more closely in touch with the family matrix as an active dynamic force in individual lives than is the case elsewhere in Britain. Likewise group therapy was readily accepted, but the dynamics were different to those elsewhere. These were not stranger groups. My first group was held in Lerwick. At the first session everyone who arrived greeted everyone else, except for one, an incomer, although her family roots had been in Shetland. The only 'stranger', she was the one who found the group hardest to integrate into.

Years previously I got together a doctor–clergy group at Powick, and I had always sought to promote dialogue between the Church and medicine. In Lerwick I organised monthly meetings with the members of the local Presbytery, and these were well attended and I believe useful. Religion in the far North is more 'down to earth' than I have often found it elsewhere. Many of the old factions and divisions which caused such bitter strife in the 19th century have now gone. It was a good group. It set me thinking about how opinion had swung in my own family. My great-great-grandfather was a staunch member of the Established Church of Scotland, being an Elder for 50 years. My great-grandfather joined the Free Church after the 'disruption' of 1843, where he also was an Elder. My grandfather followed, but he disliked public office, and sensibly remained an ordinary member of the Free Church in Lerwick for most of his life. My grandmother, who enjoyed being a reactionary, went to the Episcopalian Church, usually known as 'the English Church'. I doubt if these churches were talking to each other in those days, but in my group, Free Church, Established Church and Episcopalian ministers all met together.

The problem of alcoholism was becoming a serious issue. Some of us got together to form a steering group to address matters. Greatly increased prosperity from the coming of oil demanded quick ways of spending money, and alcohol was one of the leading contenders. In 1979, a weekend conference was held in Lerwick to address this matter (Sandison 1979). The symposium was well attended by a wide range of professionals, workers and other interested persons. The nine principal speakers included Dr Mildred Blaxter, of the Medical Research Council's unit in Aberdeen, Mr Marcus Grant, Director of the Alcohol Education Centre at the Maudsley Hospital, London, Inspector Patrick Douglas of the Northern Constabulary, and Dr Bruce Ritson from the Alcohol Resource Centre at the Royal Edinburgh Hospital, the remainder being from Shetland itself. The outcome of this conference was the formation of the Alcohol Resource Centre in Lerwick, which has grown and thrived through the years. Today it is usual to read in the local paper that most of those convicted under the drinking and driving laws have as a condition of their sentence to attend an alcohol awareness course.

After the dream about Evelyn, I recorded no other dreams until after I left Shetland. Instead, I gave my unconscious another outlet by writing novels. The hero of my first was Magnus, a Shetlander whose father dies suddenly and he decides to travel, taking his sister with him. She is only 14 years old, and acts as Magnus's intuitive function. His anima is Pallas Athene, who manifests her power both as saviour and deceiver. After many adventures Magnus, inflated after his travels, decides, that the future peace of the world lies in forming a world federation of islands. I think I was trying to bring together all the untidy and disparate parts of my own life and psyche into a coherent whole. The idea did not appeal to publishers, and *Magnus* lies today in a drawer. There is, I believe, some good writing in it which might come to life again one day. I worked on the theme of transformation, and I remain fascinated with Magnus's mischievous adolescent anima, personified by his sister. I called her Tamar, which was my great-grandmother's name. Nearly everyone in the family has, at one time or another, been drawn to know more about Tamar. For no very clear reason she carries the anima mystery for each generation. I possess her only known surviving possession, her nursing chair, so perhaps she is the great mother in the family as well. She had nine children, all of whom survived.

I wrote *Simon's Daughter* with passionate urgency in 1981. As mentioned briefly in Chapter 2, the daughter of the title was conceived during a stormy voyage across the Atlantic, and Simon did not see her until she was 14, the same age as Tamar in *Magnus*. In *Simon's Daughter* I play with time and time shifts, the meaning of chance and telepathy. The book is full of anima figures through whose world Simon was drifting. His partial solution to his life problems is a religious one, but I have never been very satisfied with it. In the last scene he watches people coming out of a church and finds that they are all the people he has ever known. I was thinking of a similar dream which I had at that time. The book was published in 1984, and is dedicated to Beth, not by name, but to 'She who gave the Fire'. It puzzled my publisher. I was at the time doing some group work for the Cistercian order. It was work which gave me an opportunity to reflect, as I had no idea where I should be going.

My search for a model for my own style of psychotherapy was reaching maturity. The years in Shetland and Aberdeen allowed me to develop and refine a way of practising group, individual and family therapy which could be realised. It was the doctor in me that felt unrealised and dissatisfied. Uncle Jack had not only travelled the islands bringing comfort and mental succour. He had delivered babies in strange places; he had removed appendixes on the kitchen tables of croft houses with a relative dropping chloroform on to the mask at his direction; he had pursued a campaign against tuberculosis with swab, slide and microscope. For long I had felt that reproductive medicine and psychiatry belonged together, a theme which I shall develop in the next chapter.

In 1978 the doctor who had been running the family planning clinics in Shetland left and no one was qualified to take on the job. My colleagues were quite happy for me to train and take this over. I went to Glasgow, and trained under Dr Wilson and her team. I brushed up on my gynaecology in Aberdeen, and was duly accepted by the National Association of Family Planning Doctors as a member. Later, I took the advanced course and qualified as an instructing doctor. I felt at last like a 'proper doctor'. Family planning was to me a very satisfying speciality. The patients were not ill; my job required precision, care, some surgical skills and was based on first principles. Decisions were made jointly between doctor and patient, and a good consultation resulted in the patient knowing that she would be protected from an unwanted pregnancy, and was thus a great dispeller of anxiety. I was glad also of the opportunity to make a direct contribution to a subject which had been at the back of my mind ever since my mother had been a supporter of Marie Stopes and her pioneering efforts in the 1920s.

My desire to extend the range of the work of healing led me to study acupuncture. I studied in London under Felix Mann. He had spent ten years in China, learned Mandarin and not only knew a vast amount about Chinese medicine, but was also an excellent teacher. Taken in its original from, acupuncture is a beautiful and exact science. A lot of mumbo-jumbo has been tacked onto it both in China and Europe, but I ignored all this. I rather liked the idea of a system which worked even though its theoretical base appeared to have no physiological or anatomical corollaries. It was like a physical psychotherapy. As in analysis, something happened but you never quite knew how. And, just as one often feels completely emotionally drained after a session with a patient, acupuncture, I found, was similarly draining. I have never practised it widely, but I found it very useful in Shetland for back pain, a common complaint there.

By the beginning of 1982 it was clear that I had to make some major decisions. Shetland needed a full-time psychiatrist, and I could not undertake that. The course at Aberdeen no longer required me on a regular basis. I could have retired and gone on living in Shetland, but I felt that I had a lot of professional life in me which was demanding an outlet. Above all, although I had many good friends there, I had been too long away from the place ever to feel that I truly belonged. It was only after I left that I began to feel that I did belong after all.

When my great-great-grandfather's diaries came to light in 1986 I started to research his life, and learned that he had been a frequent visitor to the Haa of Ollaberry in the 1820s and 1830s. The Haa houses of Tangwick and Ollaberry, 12 miles apart, formed the domain of the Cheyne brothers, John and Arthur. Christopher, my great-great-grandfather, was factor, or agent, to both. During the ten years I was working on Christopher's life I developed a great affection for him, I even had fantasies of being his reincarnation. I was able to explain the irresistible yearning which took me to the place where I was invisibly touching his life. I knew the house in Tangwick where he had lived, by then a ruin. I might have restored that, but it was too powerful a place. Perhaps one day one of my descendants will be moved to do so. It took me nearly ten years to transcribe his diaries, to research his life and to write his biography. It was published in Shetland in 1997, and launched in the very room in Tangwick where he had spent much time. It was a numinous occasion, with many people there. Pride of place went to Tina, Christopher's only surviving relative still living in Tangwick. A large lady, she sat like a queen in the middle of the gathering. That evening marked my true farewell to Shetland.

In 1982 other matters were on my mind. I was forging stronger and stronger ties with the Group Analytical Society (London), and I was, at the time, doing some worthwhile work for the Cistercians which they were anxious for me to pursue, although I had doubts about that. I had met John Guillebaud at a family planning conference who said that if I decided to come to London he would be happy for me to work at the Margaret Pyke Centre which he directed. My wife was becoming more and more remote. She joined the Roman Catholic Church. It was her choice to do so, but it created a further barrier. She left Shetland in May of that year. I agonised for weeks, looking and praying for a sign. There was no flash of light or tablets of stone, it was just that one day I knew what I had to do. I put everything up for sale except for the two cottages on the beach, including my beloved boat and my car. Beth came to Shetland that summer and stayed in the small house I owned in Lerwick. I went south and bought a flat in central London, close to the then headquarters of the Group Analytic Society. It was another exciting adventure, but something had gone for ever. I had tried to reconcile the Englishness of my mother and the unique blend of Celt and Norseman which was my father's heritage. The child of separated parents, asked which one he would wish to be with, most often will choose the one he happens to be with at the time. So it was with me. I am glad I went. I have experienced gales of one hundred miles an hour in winter. I have heard the wind screaming down from the north-west and felt the bitter sting of the hail that came with it. I have seen the great pillars of black cloud building up and up before a storm. I have gone out on a calm night and seen the northern lights, the 'merry dancers' painting the whole sky with curtains of colour. I have been to remote places where few people go. I have seen the incomparable beauty of a summer evening when it was said you could hear a bird turning over a stone a mile away across the water. I have heard the strange mournful cry of the Loon, the red-throated diver, in summer and the plaintiff honk of the whooper swan in winter. I write this with tears in my eyes. The power of Shetland exceeds that of all other islands, as any Shetlander will tell you.

CHAPTER 5

1. Groups: The Group Analytic Society and Groups with Religious and Others. LONDON 1982–1992

I saw patients in Shetland until the end of September 1982. Towards the end of October I packed some personal belongings into the back of the car and set off for Pitlochry, where I took part in the annual three-day psychotherapy conference. It was all part of my leave taking. Shetland may have been a difficult place to be in, but it is the hardest place in the world to leave. Leaving Pitlochry, I crossed the Irish sea to Belfast and drove to Portglenone, about 15 miles to the north. Portglenone is a small town which plays host to The Abbey of Our Lady of Bethlehem, the only Catholic monastery in the Province, run by Cistercians. There I met Father Stephen from Caldey and Terry Lear, a group analyst. Our objective was to run a group-dynamics workshop for the monks. This was at the height of the 'troubles', and the level of stress was very high.

I have plunged into this story of my work with religious and priests in the middle. It has a history whose roots date back to the clergy groups at Powick, and whose 'catholic connection' started with Tony ffrench-Mullen, Catholic chaplain to the Southampton hospitals, who became a patient of mine in 1971. At the moment this history is unimportant. My passage through Ireland on my way from Shetland to London was a powerful metaphor reminding me of the unhealed split in myself. In Portglenone I found myself at the very point of tension between the opposites. It was a terrifying and paralysing place, but our task as a team was to stand sufficiently far outside it so as to support the monks and help them and us to make sense of the dynamics. The town itself reflected division. Half, such as the police station and the telephone exchange, was a war zone, protected by high wire fences and armed men. The remainder of the town was preparing for the arrival of the Orangemen. Even the kerbstones were painted red, white and blue, and one of us noticed that some women in sandals had their toenails similarly adorned. Violence was never far away. A policewoman had been shot and killed by a gunman from inside the monastery's walls. There had been a car bomb and other atrocities.

The Cistercian tradition dates from the rule of St Benedict, born in 480 AD in what is now Umbria in Italy. It is a rule for group living that has survived with small modifications throughout the ages. A chapter of it is read every morning to the daily meeting of the monks. It emphasises the need to care for each other and that the care of guest and visitors comes before all else. We stayed in the guest house, which had become a refuge, with large numbers of visitors, mostly from Belfast, coming each day for rest, refreshment and counselling. Some came to just 'be there', others had been bereaved or in other ways were victims of violence. They were helped by a small group from the 35 members of the community. On Sundays up to 500 people might come, quite overwhelming the resources of the monks. It was enough for many just to come to a place where they felt the presence of God and prayer, and where they felt safe for a few hours. We had hoped that the monks would share some of their own stresses and doubts with us, but it soon became clear that this was a 'no-go' area and we became passive observers of the process. However, many of the visitors were so needy that they were happy to talk to us, or to anyone who would listen. Their belief in the power of religion was great. One woman, dipping her finger into holy water as she left, was heard to say, 'Maybe this will protect us better than the authorities.' Her son had been kidnapped the week before.

Even today, more than 17 years later, the intensity of that experience has not left me. While I was reflecting on writing this I had a terrifying dream. I was in a cathedral in Northern Ireland. There were no pews or chairs, just the bare hard stone floor. A group of the 'men of violence' was in possession. Their victims were about to be punished. A huge man in front of me had a naked victim in his arms, whom he was preparing to throw into the air so that he would crash to the stone floor. In the dream terrible injuries could be inflicted in this manner. What I was caught up in was the increasing bodily tension in the victim in the final moments before he was thrown. For a few moments I carried all the tension between North and South, Saxon and Celt, Protestant and Catholic. Mercifully I did not see the fall, but I heard the men say chillingly that the result was 'very satisfactory'. At another level, I can see that all of those conflicts are inescapable elements in my own nature. However, I remember that we asked Father Martin how he was able to reconcile his regular visits to the Maze Prison to counsel and pray with terrorists on the one hand, and his work with their victims on the other. His reply was, 'When you see two sheep, both caught on the wire, but on different sides, you try to rescue both, which side they are on becomes unimportant.' It seemed simple, put like that. My dream reminded me that, as the sheep discovered, the wire is a very dangerous place.

Terry Lear and I both have Celtic roots, and could readily resonate with the deep concern of the Portglenone monks for nature, and with the monk's inherent concern for his brother, his fierce loyalties and his distrust of strangers. It contrasts with the Judaeo-Christian tradition that has leeched the sacred out of nature and invested it in God. We found Father Bernard deeply involved in the observation of a badger sett just outside the guest-house, getting up in the night hours to see to it.

The experience in the small and large groups was both moving and humbling. Out of the community of 35, 22 elected to take part, although four more came to the large groups only. Of the remainder, there were one or two hermits who lived somewhere in the grounds and were seldom seen, which left a small number who preferred their solitude and silence to any form of group activity. We learned, as I had previously done at Caldey, how isolated and solitary many of them were. They had great difficulty in communicating with others, had fears of self-expression and self-revelation, reinforced by years of traditional habits of thinking, silence and, for most, lack of contact with the outside world. We felt that we, as a staff, had made progress, and likened our work to the first chapter of Genesis. On the first day all was void and chaos, by the fourth day, when man appears in the story, we felt that most members of the group had become aware of each other as separate people, and that the word 'I' had begun to have a meaning. On the fifth day we had the final group, and left, with a promise to return in the following year.

One does not go to a monastery just to lead a group. One goes to join a group as well. As at Caldey, we joined the life of the monks, went to their offices, shared their daily chapter meetings. I was the only Protestant in the staff group, but I was not made to feel different. It was an interesting and creative exchange of authority. By the very act of entering the monastery we were handing over our authority to the monks, but in the groups they surrendered that authority to us. Hence, mirroring, by which I mean the ability to see the whole group as a mirror of oneself, was an important dynamic.

I returned to London. It had a familiarity about it. I had known it for most of my childhood, and during the greater part of my training, and I now searched for some anchors for my professional self. I selected my flat close to the then home of the Group Analytic Society near Baker Street. In 1981, before I left Shetland, I had made a bold excursion into its inner sanctum. S.F. Foulkes, the founder of group analysis and of the Group Analytic Society and Institute, died in 1976. He died while leading a group of senior colleagues. Like all founders he had become invested by invincibility and immortality, although he had tried hard to avoid it. During the years which followed his death, the committee floundered, there were power struggles to find a successor, and an interregnum stunted growth. During the decade in which Foulkes died there was little control of membership, and many joined the Society whose connections with group work were tenuous or dubious. Some had joined for political motives.

I was aware of most of these matters through my friendship with Jane Abercrombie, who became President of the Society in 1981. From her I learned that the committee was in disarray, but at the same time adopting that dangerous stance to the effects that all was well. At least one member was about to resign, and Jane herself doubted whether she could continue her three years of chairmanship after the first year. I offered to act as facilitator for a committee 'retreat' which, rather to my surprise, was accepted. The workshop, or retreat, took place on 7 and 8 November and only two members of the committee declined to attend. We met at Elizabeth Foulkes' home for a social evening, and the next day had four sessions at the Society's rooms in Bickenhall Mansions. It took nearly all day of gathering trust for the group to be able to address the central issue, and it was not until the afternoon that the fact of Foulkes' death was mentioned. Our very reason for being together had been in danger of being still-born. Once again, I observed the dictum of 'trust the group' coming unfailingly to our aid. There was anger, disbelief, frustration, until one member said simply, 'I was there when he died.' Somehow that statement of reality liberated the group into recognition, mourning and the knowledge that it was Foulkes who had died, not the Society.

There had been talk of another similar workshop in the February following, but this never took place; indeed it did not seem appropriate after I received letters from Jane Abercrombie and Tom Hamrogue which resonated with pleasure and relief that the meeting resulted in a revival of the committee's dormant spirit. Jane spoke of my having given my 'time and skills' to 'recalcitrant material', and added that she felt 'very invigorated by the retreat' and had decided to continue her chairmanship for the full term of three years. A member who had decided to resign from the committee had changed her mind. Jane ended by saying that she thought a 'dangerous episode' in the life of the Society had been integrated and come to terms with and added, 'I shall quite look forward to telling the two people on the committee who absented themselves what a lot they missed.'

I do not claim any special talent for facilitating a 'recalcitrant group'. I find it sad and astonishing that so many groups limp along at a low level of satisfaction and achievement and at the same time deny the need for any outside help. Committees, self-help groups and the myriad so-called groups that pride themselves on what they are doing in small towns and parishes fall victim to this incestuous homeostasis.

This workshop, together with the success of the Edzell Grange group work course, made me feel that I had a home and belonged. I cannot say to this day what label I carried, or how I was seen by other members of the Society. I can only record some of the things I did in and for the Society. These gave me a sort of sense of belonging, although in many ways I have never felt that I belonged anywhere. Perhaps that is why Andrew Powell once said of me that I seemed at home wherever I was. My arrival in London intensified these feelings. I went to the January workshop of the Society as a member, where I was fortunate to be in a group run by Louis Zinkin. Nevertheless it was an uncomfortable experience. I felt ill at ease, emotionally drained and flat, and I was mourning losses which I could not verbalise. I had pursued a dream and an ideal on at least two fronts, and they had ended, as some dreams we have in sleep do, without any apparent conclusion or resolution. The dreams of sleep can be worked on and eventually understood. My waking dreams and their attempted fulfilment took several years to work through. Two years after I arrived in London I started analysis with Louis Zinkin. The process had started during the group in which fate had placed me during the Society's January workshop of 1983. I refer briefly again to this analysis in the chapter 'A Century of Psychotherapy'. The process will be interwoven into the material of this chapter also, since a personal analysis only acquires meaning when its context, the life of the analysand, is known.

In those two years, 1982–1984, I was more than once poised at the junction of opposites. In August of 1983 Beth and I went to France where we explored the glories of Chartres, relaxed under the spell of the Loire, camped in the de Sevres, paddled on the waterways of Coulon and Mauzé, and feasted on delicacies in Rouen. We discovered that we made good travelling companions, which I believe to be a fair test of a relationship. While in France I had a series of dreams about Shetland, which made me recall that when I went to Shetland in 1975 I had a series of dreams about France. Perhaps the archetype of the 'auld alliance' was surfacing. However, far from an alliance, conflict was apparent again. I was in Shetland hoping to go south, but missed the boat because I was casually chatting to friends. I missed the last train before Christmas from London to the North for the same reason. I ran after it, and could have caught it, except that it went into a tunnel...

My compensation, as always, for this state of mind was to plunge into personal and professional activities. They fall fairly neatly into four areas, the Group Analytic Society, the London Pastoral Support Group, the clinics for psychosexual disorders and family planning at the Margaret Pyke Centre, Soho, and private psychotherapeutic practice. They are not easy to separate, and they will, in this narrative, continually interweave and overlap. I believe I contributed something to each of these fields, and in the process I learned much about the human condition and about myself.

The Group Analytic Society was gradually finding its identity. Its maturity was still a long way off in 1983, and I had the interesting but difficult task of living and working with it during its growth pains. I formed a sub-committee to consider categories of membership, the professional and personal qualifications required for being accepted into membership, and the host of practical details needed to make the process work. We worked for a year on this, meeting for a whole day once a month, and our recommendations were adopted, and remain largely in place today. It was an important group for me, as it gave me a sense of belonging. Otherwise, it was unremarkable, and any more detail would sound pedestrian. My involvement did lead to my being elected to the committee of the Society. It was the committee which I had led in the crucial workshop two years earlier, although its membership had changed to some extent. The dynamics of committees as a genus are quite depressing. Their *raison d'être* is agendas and decisions. The committee of the GA Society was always trying to look at its dynamics, but never quite succeeded in doing so. When Dennis Brown became President we spent a day each year 'in retreat' at his country cottage in Berkshire. The idea was that we should look at some of our own group dynamics, but of course we never did. Curiously enough, it never occurred to anyone to invite a facilitator from outside. There might have been an archetypal fear of attempting this. Rider Haggard's *She* (1998) had attained eternal life by bathing in the fire deep inside a mountain in central Africa, but when she repeated the experience she shrivelled and died. I was also a member and had as much responsibility as the others, but perhaps I too was caught up in the dynamic of homeostasis.

In 1987 Elizabeth Foulkes, who had edited the Society's Bulletin since her husband's death in 1976, decided to retire from this position, and I took it over, and continued until 1993. I was taking over an organ directly descended from Foulkes' Group Analysis International Panel and Correspondence (GAIPAC), which he started in 1967 in order to establish dialogue between a wide international network of friends and correspondents who had followed his work closely. I tried to follow the same tradition. However, an editor has to work with what he receives. Over the years I had a large number of reports, letters, reviews and comments. They were nearly all written in the relaxed, informal and often humorous style which is denied to the authors of papers for scientific journals. Sadly, from time to time I had obituary notices, all of which were written with great sensitivity, a declaration of the bonding love which existed between members. In my first issue dated January 1988, I recorded the deaths of Prue Skynner and Richard Finlayson. I had worked with Prue and Robin Skynner two years earlier at a group analytic workshop for bishops and their wives, while Richard had been a most committed member of the working party on membership which I had chaired five years earlier. Rita Lynn's tribute to Prue was written in the form of a letter to her, and is among the most beautiful and sensitive obituaries I have come across. These tributes made me realise, more than anything else, the invisible bonds of affection and regard which most of the members of the GA Society enjoy, and I felt at last part of that fellowship.

Five years later, I had retired to my present home in Herefordshire, and it was time to hand over the editorship. Anne Harrow and Sheila Thomson not only took this on, but they have increased the size and scope of the Bulletin, now called 'Group Analytic Contexts'. They continue a tradition to this day which Foulkes started over 30 years ago. The issue of September 1998 contained several accounts of the Study Day of May 1998 at which the centenary of Foulkes' birth was commemorated. After the annual Foulkes lecture and a median group, the members of the study day met a panel of seven of the most senior members of the Society, all of whom had known him. The account was written up by Teresa Howard, and I was intrigued to find that, even among that senior group, mourning for the founder was still a disturbing issue. There was a lot of personal reminiscence by the panel, until they got on to the death instinct. Towards the end of the discussion a member of the audience asked whether the GA movement had finally mourned its founder. He had actually been talking about the recent death of Barbara Dick, who had been a member of the committee whose 'retreat' I had led 17 years earlier, so mourning was high on his agenda. Dennis Brown responded by saying, 'I've always had the feeling that Foulkes dying in a group was difficult. We never met and worked it through. Maybe today?' Astonishingly, the very member who had said in the 1981 group 'I was there' and released us into a true mourning, then said, 'We never got together to talk about it. We managed to foul it up.' The process of giving a great man a decent burial is not only long and difficult, but he is liable to be either forgotten or reviled before it can be completed. Nevertheless, this made uncomfortable reading. Perhaps, after all, I should have held that second workshop with the committee, or even a third, but, as Jung so often reminded us, processes which are deeply rooted in the unconscious have their own time agenda.

This chapter commenced with my visit to Portglenone in 1982. I have apparently digressed by writing about the survival of the GA Society after the death of Foulkes. However, much of my work with the clergy over many years has been to do with survival. Indeed, I have sometimes wondered whether the Christian Church has ever come to terms with the death of Christ. It seems so intent on eternally mourning the suffering and death of its founder that it has a permanent sense of isolation and failure. Certainly this was how I perceived hospital chaplains and many parish priests in my early years in psychiatry. The staff–clergy group which I formed in 1961 was also a response to the survival of individual priests in the face of the general loosening of moral codes and social cohesion. When it came to mental illness, some of them were still adherent to the idea that sin and sexual deviance led to insanity. The group work was directed for the first year in working through these assumptions. This stage was not without casualties, and one member felt that he had to leave the ministry because he could not reconcile his new-found insights with the teaching of the Church. I believe he managed to come to terms with this through his bishop, and that he remained in the Church. Nevertheless it was a sign that although groups may help with holding and bonding, they also exercise a powerful dynamic effect on some individuals. It was about this time that I was asked to see a man whose marriage was on the rocks. Those who referred him wrote to me as a 'Christian psychiatrist', with the implication that I would make the patient see the error of his ways and return to a spent marriage. It gave me the opportunity to declare that I was a psychiatrist and a Christian, and that it was as a psychiatrist that I saw my patients, and this is still my position.

Today I reflect that my wish to connect psychiatry and religion may have been rooted in deeper feelings about the nature of disturbance of the mind. For centuries the Church had looked after the insane. The clergy, if they had an attitude towards their charges, would have seen them as having a sickness of the soul. In broad terms, after the reforms of the poor law in the 19th century, there was a vacuum resulting in the medical profession taking over the care and treatment of the insane. Inevitably insanity became an illness, most probably a disease of the brain. It does make me wonder sometimes whether the mentally ill have got the best deal from ending up in the care of the medical profession. Put another way, many doctors were unwilling to shed their image as 'proper doctors', and use words instead of drugs.

As I mentioned at the beginning of this chapter, I met Tony ffrench-Mullen in 1971 in Southampton, who became a patient, and we worked together analytically for four years. After the war, most of which he had spent as a prisoner in Germany, having been shot down in one of the early bombing raids, he joined the Cistercian monks at Caldey. The rule of St Benedict insists on stability, meaning that once you join a monastery you stay there with that group until you die. Tony was too big for Caldey and he left. I discovered that those who left this monastery became non-persons, as nobody in the order seemed to care or enquire what happened to them. Indeed one of the events that led to my working professionally with the Caldey community in 1979 was the defection of their abbot. This had happened about two years earlier and no one knew where he was, nor seemed to care. Perhaps I should have been warned by that attitude.

I was drawn to Caldey by both conscious and unconscious forces, of which the latter were by far the most potent. The most immediate was my counter-transference to Tony, compounded by my curiosity and need to know more about the place where he had spent some 20 years of his life. It was a relatively small island, a centre of religious faith and practice. These in combination are among the most powerful forces of fatal attraction I know. I also had an inner hankering to live the life of a monk, and the chance to do this by proxy, so to speak, came in 1979. Tony had asked me to conduct a group dynamics workshop for some of the parishioners of the parish to which he moved after leaving

Southampton. Just before we started, Father Stephen from Caldey, the only monk there who had kept in touch with Tony, arrived. I liked Stephen, although sadly he has been one of the very few people with whom I have fallen out, and we did so much later with bitter and uncharitable feelings, at least on my part. At that time, however, he had a story to tell. The present-day Cistercians have grown out of the Trappist tradition, and although the Rule provided a good model for organised living, it is a life without sharing. Stephen was made acutely aware of this, and wrote to me later, as follows:

> Eighteen months ago I talked to our community about our interpersonal relationships, having been shocked and distressed to discover in myself a profound ignorance of two of the brethren who had died. I had lived with them for more than thirty years but I knew scarcely anything about them, apart from the usual relatively unimportant details of their backgrounds, education and monastic upbringing. Voltaire's indictment came home to me with a vengeance; monastic communities are groups of men who live together without loving each other and die without missing each other. It is still a terrible and terribly real indictment.

Over a period of three years I conducted two workshops a year at Caldey. Each lasted three days, and I managed to arrange for two small groups each day during that time. What had been happening at Caldey was more than Stephen's perception of a community of men who 'lived together without loving each other'. A religious panic had seized them on realising that not only had two members of the community died, but that the whole community might die. They were an ageing group, new members were not arriving as they once did. They were a depressed collection of individuals. They had, it seemed to me, plunged into the contemplative life without realising that, in the words of Thomas Merton (1961), 'Before you start thinking about contemplation you have to recover your basic natural unity' (p.16).

One cannot work in an orthodox group analytic way with monks, although I believe I never lost sight of group analytic principles. They compensated for their isolation from one another by the fantasies they had of others. Herman was a Belgian, and a big man, physically and spiritually. He didn't come to the early meetings, so I suggested that they should ask him. 'Oh, no, we don't want him here, he will only talk about God all the time!' Herman did come, a very large and rather high chair was imported to support his great frame, so that he looked like a patriarch. He did not 'talk about God'. He talked about love. He looked over to one of the other members and boomed, 'If I tell you that I love you, I mean "I love you".' The exchange of such direct feelings terrified the group; no wonder they had tried to exclude him. So we inevitably progressed to sexuality, and from there to the feminine.

'How can we talk about the feminine without there being a woman in the group?' was the first comment. Finding the feminine in themselves was an experience they had once had, but lost. Each member had a history, all had had mothers, all had suppressed and projected the image on to the Virgin Mary, to whom the Cistercians have a special dedication. I think I did manage to achieve quite a lot. The community changed in many ways. For example, at the daily meetings in the Chapter House they formerly sat in rows, like an old-fashioned schoolroom. They changed this to a circle and decided that it was a good way to work. They acknowledged each other's presence with a slight raising of the hand as they passed in the cloister or wherever. In the Chapter House the abbot had hitherto read a chapter of the Rule each day. Now they took it in turns, and commented, initiating a short discussion. Stephen wrote: 'There is now in our Community frequent discussion, a frankness, honesty and calmness which would not have been possible 18 months ago.' The monastery survived, and from occasional references in the Press, I note that it is alive and active today.

Islands exact tribute, and I should have learned that lesson from my experience in Shetland, but my odyssey was not over, and I was still to suffer as Odysseus himself did. I made placatory gifts to the island community which weakened my conscious control over my life. Unfortunately Father Stephen, who was my correspondent and link with the community over the years, exploited my goodwill in a quite astonishing and unprofessional manner. He too was in the grip of unconscious forces he did not understand, and these were never resolved between us. The circumstances which led to my breaking my connection with Caldey are not relevant to this book, and I have no wish to pursue them here, as they involve many people alive today. But I suffered the same fate as Tony and the ex-abbot, I departed in haste, and was seen by the community as the sinner. In 1988 Beth met the ex-abbot in London by chance. She felt that he was still paying tribute. Stephen and I at one time had a profuse correspondence, but, looking at it again, it is clear that there was always an unbridgeable gulf in meaning between us. It reminded me that Jung and the Dominican priest Father Victor White also had a very long correspondence, that they never reached a rapprochement, and they fell out rather bitterly after they met face to face. Mercifully, they managed some healing when White was dying, but it was rather late. Dominicans are different from Cistercians. For one thing, the Cistercians of Caldey are still on their enchanted island.

It took me a long time to work all this out. At one time I wrote about my group and other work with them with uncritical enthusiasm. Now that I am no longer in thrall to the community and to the island, it has been difficult to write about the many good personal experiences I had during my visits. I know I could never have lived there. Like Tony, I felt too big for the place and that was the only way that I managed to escape. The monks at Caldey had seen me as their saviour-therapist, and when I declared my humanness and sanity by severing my connections with them they saw it as a sign of defection. It is hard for most of us to live with paradox; it is almost impossible for monks.

At about the time of the disruption from Caldey I was invited to join the London Pastoral Support Scheme (the Scheme) as a consultant. The Scheme had been started by Robin Skynner about seven years previously. In true Anglican style, it operated in layers, which they called tiers. The third tier existed in the parishes, and consisted of groups run by leaders trained in group dynamics. They had been trained in the second tier groups, which also were the supervision groups for all the group leaders of the third tier. The first tier was the consultants, who were supposed to be four, two senior and two others. Of those 'others', I saw little, but on the whole the scheme worked well.

I was glad that much of the work of persuading members of the Church that small groups were a valid way of working had already been done. The clergy in general are suspicious of them, although Catholics are more at ease than Protestants. Parish priests who have only a small congregation fail to exploit the small group potential of this situation. Moses was more percipient nearly 4000 years ago, when he divided his people into hundreds and into tens. Our term *deacon* describes the priest who looked after ten people. When St Bernard, in the Middle Ages, founded the monastery of Citeaux he did so with 12 monks. They were the first Cistercians.

My task was the supervision and growth of a group of priests and parish workers, and we met as a slow open group for seven years. I witnessed in this group some of the forces which surface in a group composed of people who, as it were, lived close to God. God, or a spiritual force, is always somewhere in every group, and the same is true in individual therapy. Here, God was more evident, and if God was there, the devil had to be as well. The following situation in my group demonstrated this rather well.

M. had been in therapy for many years with E., a member of the supervision group. A new member, D., joined this group who, unknown either to me or to E., was preparing M. to train for the ministry. When M. got to hear of this she became intensely angry and paranoid, believing that her 'case' would be discussed in the supervision group thus prejudicing D. against her. She withdrew from E.'s group and D. felt that he should withdraw from the supervision group, which fortunately he did not. The point is that M.'s ghost raged unseen round our group for weeks, resulting in splitting and consequent paralysis to the work of the group. The summer recess was approaching and we had resolved nothing. At that point, D. had a tremendous outburst against M., his pupil, almost like one possessed. It had the remarkable effect of healing the split between himself and E., and allowed the group to resume its work. What had happened? Certainly the ghost of M. had been laid, but we also realised that we had needed this unseen spirit to prise us out of the comfort which often in a slow open group obscures deep and destructive passions. There were, for example, aspects of E.'s counter-transference to M. which had not been explored and which had remained hidden until D. joined the group. Thus it was D. who was the 'third force', but having raised this force it became attached to the group matrix, becoming personified as M. who became a powerful metaphor for destruction. The victim was E. who, like Pygmalion, had created M. in his own image, and to whom D.'s revelations together with the fantasies of the group about M. were a bitter blow. In accepting this he became released from feelings of obligation to M. which had lasted for over 20 years, and could allow her to pursue her own way, which she did in the ministry.

M. was then able to return to her own group, where she acknowledged her deviant behaviour. Two weeks later her group conductor was tragically killed in a road traffic accident. He was not only mourned greatly in her group, but also in our supervision group, as he was known by and loved by us all. We reflected that his sudden death appeared meaningless, but, if he had to go, the timing of it could not have been better. We rejoiced that he had lived to share with us our faith in the healing ability of the group matrix.

Ernest was a retired priest who was a member of this group, and also in therapy with me. The group knew of the latter, and I never felt that either process hampered either the group or our therapy. One of the members of Ernest's group was pregnant, and after she gave birth she decided she wanted to bring the baby to the group. After some hesitation the group accepted this, and the child added a new dimension to the matrix. He resonated with the mood of the group, and gave members cues. Breast feeding raised their awareness of a host of issues: dependency, nurturing, privacy, and above all, was the child a member of the group? They took Winnicott's view, that 'there is no such thing as a baby, there is only a mother and baby'. Something else occurred. The Judaeo-Christian faith emphasises the spiritual power and wisdom of the child: 'And a little child shall lead them.' The Christ child, in uncanonical stories, could perform miracles at a very early age. It is reminiscent of the infant Hermes, who stole the celestial cattle by cunning when he was but three days old. A mother once brought a baby to one of my own groups, and we were much enriched by the experience.

The London Diocesan Support Scheme came to an end in 1991. It was originally conceived after meetings between Hewlett Thompson, then Bishop of Willesden, Joy Thompson, Robin Skynner and Prue Skynner, the last three being group analysts. The Scheme lasted for 17 years, starting as a 'cottage industry' and gradually becoming absorbed into the bureaucracy of the Church. The problem was that although Diocesan House wanted to take control of all pastoral schemes, there was nobody available who had a sufficient understanding of group dynamics to do so. It is not particularly rewarding to study the dynamics of death by starvation. The fact that it took off in the first place was owing to the dedication and enthusiasm of a small group of people. All four had left the scene by 1990. We appealed to the London bishops, I held discussions with David Hope, then Bishop of London. Brian Snowden and I put up a number of alternative suggestions, but they were lost in the bureaucratic machine. It is more profitable to look at the dynamics of clergy and parish worker support in the wider context of the Anglican Church. There is a widespread confusion of thinking which mixes up support and supervision groups with therapy. When Brian and I wrote to all the London bishops, the only considered reply came from the Bishop of Stepney, who concluded: 'It is irritating that clergy keep on asking for more pastoral support but then reject the schemes which are offered to them.' Nevertheless, there is a great hunger among the clergy and others for more support, and it is not entirely true that they reject opportunities. In September 1991 Brian Snowden and I ran a one-day group dynamics workshop and attracted 37 applicants. It was hard work and took up a lot of our time partly because we had to organise the whole thing ourselves without support from the Professional Ministry Committee.

I still work as a consultant to St Luke's Hospital, but there is no opportunity for group work. In my retirement I look with sadness at the struggling inadequacies of the local parish groups, which could be so much more dynamic and effective with a supervisor. Such reflections are not profitable, and I prefer to cast my mind back to my experience of conducting my group over seven years. We discovered in that group that the more you reveal and acknowledge your humanity, the greater your spiritual power becomes. I would wish to dedicate my thoughts on these matters to Ernest Chitty. His family had its roots in the rich earth of Sussex, and everything he did reflected his spirituality. He was in the group almost to its end, and for the last three years of his life we worked together in individual therapy. On the last day of his life we had our session in the morning, and, for some reason, I wondered whether I would see him again. He lived alone, and that evening, as he was saying his Office at home, he died. I could only give thanks for all that I had learned from him. I think his daughter knew the strength of our relationship, and we still correspond. I value those rather frustrating years, but even if the only reward had been to meet Ernest I should have felt enriched. Fortunately, there was much more.

CHAPTER 6

2. Psychosexual Medicine, Family Planning and the Healing Process in Groups. LONDON 1982–1992

In London I was organising my professional life in a way which must be unusual for a psychiatrist. All psychiatrists have started their careers by training at medical school. Even at the most enlightened schools there is not much commitment to psychodynamics. I suspect that most psychiatrists yearn to be 'proper doctors', and they achieve this by an inflated adherence to the medical model. In so doing they lose touch with the patient as a human being possessing a mind, or whose mind has been stunted or scarred, or whose capacity for good relationships is impaired. The patient becomes a 'case' characterised by symptoms that add up to a diagnosis. With almost computer-like precision the appropriate drug treatment or regime follows.

I struggled with that desire to be a 'proper doctor' for over 40 years, and at first the temptation to follow the medical model in psychiatry was strong. The thing which saved me in the end was never losing sight of my patient as an individual, as someone to whom good relationships and the quality of his life mattered more than anything else. I have already described in earlier chapters how I searched for a model which would bring together the two psychiatries, organic and dynamic. I had believed it was in my grasp when I worked with LSD as a tool for psychotherapy. It became discredited as much by my own profession as by the pressures arising from the street use of LSD.

The beginnings of a solution came during my years in the North, and were honed up when I got to London. The ten years in London were the most satisfying of my whole career. Its components were my slow open group, my private practice in individual psychotherapy, and the clinics for psychosexual medicine and family planning at the Margaret Pyke Centre. My professional 'homes' and resource were the Group Analytic Society (London), and The National Association of Family Planning Doctors, now a faculty of the Royal College of Gynaecology. This at first sight appears to be a perpetuation of the split in myself, but reproductive medicine and psychiatry are first cousins. Freud found the connection inescapable, and many psychiatrists have specialised in psychosexual medicine and family therapy.

For me the connection had existed from my earliest years. I was the only child, and there was at one time talk of a 'little sister', but she never came. Then, one day when I was about seven, the high-wheeled pram, which had long stood empty, was given away. Our neighbours had five children, most other families we knew had only one. I puzzled over the difference, thinking that those parents had some almost super-human control over their instincts. Then I heard talk of 'birth control', in hushed tones. I discovered that my mother secretly had a copy of *Married Love* by Marie Stopes. I read it secretly and I never told anyone what I had learned. Matters came into the open when she organised a meeting in the town at which Stopes herself was the principal speaker. But I never dared ask any questions, or, if I did, I was received with silence or an embarrassed evasion. My curiosity was far wider than a desire to know what went on in the parents' bedroom. I knew how it was done, and had an inkling of how you stopped what it was that they did from making a baby, but the question was, why?

My childhood, sheltered as it was from much contact with working-class families, shielded me also from knowing what Marie Stopes spent her life fighting for. When I got to King's College Hospital I saw the plight of the women of Camberwell whose whole reproductive lives centred around child-bearing, poverty, fear of pregnancy, and the morbidity which resulted from their frequent child-bearing. It was then that I knew what Marie Stopes had been about, and how thinly spread the message was, even in 1938. One quarter of all the admissions to the gynaecological wards of King's were believed to be owing to the result of a 'back-street' abortion which had ended in injury or infection. The out-patient clinics were crowded with patients in unspeakable discomfort as the result of excessive child-bearing and poverty. Despite this, I do not recall any patient being instructed in contraception, nor did we have any tuition in the subject. Abortion, of course, was subject to a total taboo. We only learned about 'miscarriage', and how to prevent it, so that, presumably, the woman could add to her already large family.

Marie Stopes was, as one might expect, a most unusual woman. Her friend Mary Stocks wrote of her (reported by Box 1967): 'She was compassionate, headstrong, tactless, public-spirited, humourless, intellectually distinguished and wholly lacking in aesthetic taste. I count it a privilege to have known her. I remember her with affection, and I shall never forget her' (p.9). She opened the first birth control clinic in Britain in Holloway, North London, in March 1921. The advice and supply of contraceptives was free, being financed by herself and her husband, Humphrey Roe. She proceeded to launch a campaign which started with the publication of *Married Love* in 1918, which ran to at least 26 editions, followed by a series of books and pamphlets. In 1921, soon after her first clinic opened, she held a meeting at Queen's Hall in the West End of London, attended by a large audience and addressed by a galaxy of distinguished people. Today we dwell obsessively on the miseries of people in other countries, ignoring evils at home. Most people were as anxious to deny the squalor produced by ignorance and poverty in 1920 as they are today. Marie Stopes spoke at that meeting of a girl of 20 who was pregnant for the sixth time, having had all the previous pregnancies terminated by her mother. Other speakers spoke of even more distressing cases.

The Catholic Church watched these events with its characteristic uneasiness, but did not openly oppose the campaign. This was left to a Catholic doctor, Halliday Sutherland, who wrote a book condemning Marie Stopes' work. He accused her of 'exposing the poor to experiments', and based his criticism on Professor Anne Louise McIlroy, who described her use of the vaginal pessary as 'the most harmful method of which I have had experience'. Stopes sued for libel, and McIlroy gave evidence in strong support of Dr Halliday. After the libel action, in which the jury found against her, she discovered that Professor McIlroy was actually fitting the kind of pessaries which she had condemned in the High Court. Characteristically, she decided to check this by carefully disguising herself as a poor woman and attending the Royal Free Hospital. 'Three hours later I left the hospital with the vaginal rubber cap, which had been advised and inserted in me by Professor McIlroy.'

The libel action then went to the Appeal Court, which found in Stopes' favour, and finally to the House of Lords, which found against her. The publicity resulting from these hearings was an enormous boost to her work. Her academic background lay in natural sciences, geology and anthropology. For two years before her death in 1958 she was working on a birth control pill. It has even been suggested that we might never have had the pill if it had not been for her pioneer work. The institutional prejudices which she fought are still with us today, but in different form. The insistence of academic psychiatry on a strict medical model and its dependence on theories of brain chemistry and on the pharmaceutical industry overlook the fact that there are probably at least ten times as many people who could benefit from psychotherapy as those who are being treated with anti-psychotic drugs. Yet psychotherapy in the NHS remains, as Holmes has said (1998), 'the Cinderella of Cinderellas'.

I have already argued that the modern psychiatric institution is not necessarily any better than the good mental hospital of 50 or more years ago. Indeed it could be postulated that psychotic patients and long-stay patients have lost a great deal by the closure of most mental hospitals. In the field of family medicine and contraception there cannot be any doubt that the vast majority of women, their children and their families have benefited enormously by the spread of family planning to all branches of society. Even in the 1920s the means were there but the desire and the desirability to apply it were absent. One learns in psychoanalysis that resistances are there for a purpose, they protect the patient from being overwhelmed by unconscious contents. Similar ideas were, and to a lesser extent are still, promulgated about contraception. The feared catastrophe is to do with the fear of rampant sexual activity, especially among the young. We delude ourselves if we argue that we are worried about teenage pregnancy rates. Nobody, apart from some dedicated workers in the field, is much concerned about this. However, there is an outcry if the proper instruction of young people in sexual physiology and contraception is proposed. There may be a deeper fear, that the universal practice of contraception will lead to an alarming population fall. Almost all the most basic and powerful biological drives are directed towards breeding success in every species on earth. The practice of abortion is, of course, closely linked to these ideas, and has been medically tabooed since Hippocrates.

As a young doctor in training a clinic patient came one day to tell me she was pregnant and unmarried. She was in her late 30s and held an important professional post. She was in great distress, and yet, in 1947, I had to tell her that abortion was not possible in this country. I discussed it with my chief, but nothing could be done. I saw her twice more and I had to give the same answer. She offered me money. I have always felt that I let that patient down, but I could not have acted differently without seriously endangering my professional career. Today, in almost every clinic, she would be offered an abortion under the 1967 Abortion Act. What has changed?

I have described the 20th century as the century of psychoanalysis, and most would agree that this is one way of describing it. Many Freudian terms, such as 'the unconscious', 'Freudian slip', 'sublimation' and 'repression' have passed into the language. Novels use the language and the discoveries of Freud and Jung, biographers apply psychodynamic insights into their treatment of their subjects, others look at literature in psychoanalytic terms. Although both 'ego' and 'id' are in the dictionary, one hears the former far more frequently in everyday speech. Despite the claim that the 20th century raised people's awareness of their unconscious processes and motives, the reverse has proved to be the case. Even Jung, who spent many years studying the unconscious, declared that you could have too much of it. The very power of analytic revelations, particularly, for example, those of Melanie Kline, produced an opposite response. Both Freud and Jung battled against the strict cultural mores of their time. We have now discarded most of them and this has led us further into difficulties. Lacking boundaries of social behaviour and the loss of rites of passage leave people at the mercy of primitive unconscious elements which catch them unawares. One result of this is the persistence of outmoded responses. In the words and utterances of the media all pregnancies, especially if the woman is well-known or famous, are happy events. All the Royal marriages of the last 50 years were 'made in heaven', and were given an archetypal fairy-tale feel to them. These very expectations helped to doom most of them.

We do not have to look only in high places for confirmation. Recently I was talking to a nurse who has decided to leave her hospital after 20 years and train for the Ministry. When she told her colleagues that she was leaving, one said 'So, you're going to be a mother!', and another, 'Oh lovely, I didn't know you were pregnant!' I commented that the only difference between these responses and those which would have been made 40 years ago lay in the fact that her predecessors would have said something like, 'Oh! Who's the lucky man you're going to marry?' However, the difference is crucial. Quite unconsciously, this lady's friends had suppressed the need for the rite of passage, i.e. marriage, but had retained the age-old reason for a woman leaving any profession.

Paediatricians still speak of the milestones of childhood. Yet the old markers along that road which children travel during their growth towards maturity have been removed. We gain inner strength from reflecting on and celebrating those milestones. We may think that the old rite known as the Churching of Women is now archaic and inappropriate, although I am sure that every woman today still gives some kind of silent thanks after she has been safely delivered of her child. In other cultures it is good to hear that these rites still continue. A friend recently returned from India where he had witnessed at a Hindu temple a ceremony in which the child was brought along with the family. There he or she receive their first solid food. Sadly, the decline of religious practice has led to the loss of most of our rites of passage. But this is not the only reason for this change. The turbulent century of which we have just witnessed the close led to a belief that the ways of the past needed to be abandoned. This has resulted in identification with the chaos from which we have been striving to escape. The innocence of childhood, elevated to such heights by the Victorians, is now thought of as a disadvantage. The segregation of the sexes in adolescence, practised in many cultures, and common in our own until recently, has all but disappeared. Sexual differentiation is played down, perhaps again in response to earlier notions that the sexes were 'opposite'. We are left with the inescapable events of birth and death. Death has remained such a taboo that it is inevitable that the existence of and the phenomenon of birth has been elevated and idealised.

Loss of tradition creates a psychological and cultural vacuum. It is likely to be filled, in our present age, by government planning and regulation. It could be argued that the system of national testing of the educational attainments of

2. PSYCHOSEXUAL MEDICINE, FAMILY PLANNING...

children from an early age is an attempt at substitution for rites of passage. It would be as difficult to equate them as it is to compare a modern housing estate with an ancient village that has grown up over hundreds of years. Examinations and tests are competitive, but every child can be entered for the appropriate rite of passage and pass, so to speak. Furthermore, the tests are the same for both sexes, which extinguishes the age-old distinction between the sexes from puberty onwards. Nevertheless, these educational milestones are accepted because there is nothing else. It is not the only aspect of modern life that has been devalued and demythologised in this way.

Not only has birth become idealised, the mother herself has been elevated to the status of a Madonna. The Madonna complex decrees that the woman be pure and unsullied and that her baby must be perfect, just as the biblical Madonna was a virgin and her Child was perfect man.

It follows from preceding paragraphs that the ability to give birth has become almost the only surviving icon for creating an adult identity. If you do away with Christening, Confirmation, Marriage and their associated ceremonies, if the great festivals of Christmas, Easter and Whitsun have lost their religious meaning, there is not much left except having a baby. In psychodynamic terms, it is as if all the archetypal power of several rites of passage has been poured into a single icon. It is difficult otherwise to account for the extra-ordinary lengths to which infertile women will go in order to achieve a pregnancy.

In my generation most of my contemporaries, as children, knew that they had 'come from their mother's tummies'. How they got in there in the first place was never discussed. Consequently there was plenty of scope for fantasy and mental speculation concerning this matter. In psychoanalytic language, the parents' bedroom was a forbidden room, to enter there led to the grave penalty of the loss of innocence, a re-enactment of the Garden of Eden theme. A great many, if not the majority of, children today are denied this developmental process, and it will be interesting to follow the responses of the next generation of analysts to this. Of equal interest is what will be the psychological consequences for children whose conception was not the result of the sexual union of his or her parents. There is an old belief that happiness and prosperity in children comes from their conception during a loving and mutually satisfying sexual relationship between the parents. The issue is compounded by the dilemma of the couple who may or may not feel compelled to reveal the true state of their children's origins to them. I have professionally come across more than one woman whose children were not her husband's, she having secretly received donor sperm from a sperm bank. No one knows of this and the secret is likely to remain. The medico-legal aspects of this are outside the scope of this book. Again the psychodynamic consequences for the children of such an event have yet to be explored.

Freud has been much criticised for blaming all our psychological ills on errors and deviations in sexual development. Today it is difficult to give this sort of judgement a precise value. Sex and death remain the two great taboos of our time. One's patients help to put this in perspective, and one springs to mind. She was a university student and 20 years old. We worked together in psychotherapy for about two years. When it came to the last session she said: 'I suppose it's all been to do with sex.' I was taken aback, as sex *per se* had almost never been overt in her material. Looking back, I see her statement as a recognition that she had eaten of the fruit of sexual knowledge almost without knowing it through the transference. She had reached this goal through symbol and metaphor that are the tools of psychotherapy.

Once a taboo has been stripped of its mystery, it loses its place as something to be reflected on and studied so that one can arrive at an attitude towards it. This is specially true of abortion. In the years following the 1967 Act I was asked to see a great many women with a view to complying with the conditions of the Act. In almost all cases the distress of the patient was great, and I was able to comply with her wish. But, except in rare cases, I was denied the chance to work with the patient on the dynamic aspects of what she was undertaking. I seldom saw her partner, and very few ever came back after the operation. Inevitably, women who have had an abortion are left with an unresolved or partly resolved unconscious residue which may surface in later relationships, often in disguise. This I discovered in my work at the clinic for psychosexual disorders. In the same way, the loss of marriage as a rite of passage means for many couples that marriage is an irrelevance. The question remains as to how and where this deep-seated archetype of the mystery of the marriage ceremony will surface in their future.

At about the time I started work at the Margaret Pyke Centre I had a dream about a family, perhaps my family, who have survived the ice-age by living in a cave. I can see the melting edge of the retreating ice. The family are emerging from their cave, wearing bright colours. Lest I should get too excited about this dream, I dreamt the next night about a very beautiful young man who was being crucified upside down. A woman was floating over him from time to time, brushing her sexual hair against his. He is expecting death soon.

I had a strong feeling at the time that I had lived through an emotional ice-age. I think the second dream was a warning against getting too inflated. I was approaching 70 years of age, and the time had come to find some personal stability and a model which would align with my inner doctor-image. My work in family planning, in which I acted as locum to the Centre, fulfilled at last my need to live out, at least for a few years, the image of a doctor which I had carried with me for over 50 years. Soho was and is, to me, as it has been to many others, a fascinating place. I devoured Judith Summers' delightful history of the place she describes as the last remaining village in London's West End (Summers 1989).

The Margaret Pyke Centre was at that time located in the Soho Hospital for Women, but sadly its last remaining wards were closed not long after I arrived. It was indeed tragic to see this beautiful 18th century building deteriorate, its roof leaking and paint crumbling – a symbol of the neglect of tradition and excellence which characterise the bureaucratic machine which runs the health service. In the first chapter I wrote about my desire to understand the female psyche at the very beginning of my career in psychiatry. Part of this need had its roots in my explorations as a child into the mysteries of reproduction and birth. Birth *control* had unconscious overtones about the ability to separate sexual activity from procreation. Here, in Soho Square, this had been perfected with due regard to the scientific, human and emotional needs of women. I say women, because very few men ever came to family planning clinics.

It was estimated that the population of Soho increased by about 80,000 on every working day. Entertainment and the media were over-represented and formed a substantial part of the clientele of the clinic. As a major teaching centre it provided a complete range of options in birth control, including the 'morning-after' pill and menopausal counselling and therapy. Research was undertaken with new methods of contraception. It was a happy place. However, it was not until I started locum work in the clinics of Bloomsbury and Camden Town that I saw the kind of patients that Marie Stopes had dedicated her life to. In the multicultural society which London had become, an interpreter was sometimes needed. The difference was that these were women who no longer came secretly, were no longer overburdened with poverty and excessive child bearing. There were still tragic stories, but I was convinced that a tremendous change for the better had taken place. I found it deeply satisfying work. I had carried on a tradition derived not only from my father-uncle, but now from my mother.

My mother was then over 90 years of age and nearing the end of her life. In those last years we had many conversations which cemented the links and bonds between us which had lain dormant since my childhood. If she had not lived so long we would never have had that privilege. It seemed that at last she truly saw me as an adult, and was able to drop the defences with which she sustained her image as the happily married and contented woman. She spoke of my father's jealousy, and how he wanted her all to himself, of her sense of failure as a mother, of her feelings of defeat and exhaustion. She several times referred to the time when I was 16 and she had been in a depressed state for nearly three years. I said simply 'Mother, when are you going to get better?', and she then knew that she could. At the time this happened I had just started analysis with Louis Zinkin, and he made much of this statement.

There was something otherworldly about those conversations. She would tell me about her childhood, so that I began to understand the beginnings of her neurosis. The few years after she 'came out' at 18 until she met my father, and the years from 60 to 90, were the happiest of her life. And she still had dreams from which I understood her compassion for the deprived and the poor. She would go to the old slums of Waterloo in her dreams, where she visited an old man without food or fuel in a cottage with bare rooms. Sometimes in her dreamier moments she would speak of imaginary telephone calls from drug addicts, or men desperate for help. I began to define more clearly my desire and ability to work with depressed patients. They were privileged hours which we spent together, and perhaps few sons or daughters have that unique opportunity. After her 96th birthday she failed in health and died a month later, in March 1985. She is buried just outside the entrance of the church she had known and loved for over 50 years. I heard nothing from her for several weeks and then I had a dream that she was sitting on top of her grave and saying that she loved to sit there, where she could listen to the hymns from the church. Perhaps she did.

My regular clinic at the Margaret Pyke was one for psychosexual and marital problems. It was depressing work, with a lot of referrals of men in middle life with sexual dysfunction. Probably today some of these would be seen in a medical rather than a psychiatric setting. I had to do the best I could, which was often less than I would have wished. Most of the difficulties which arise in marital cases seemed to me to arise from lack of communication between the couple. They had either ceased to relate emotionally and verbally, or had never done so. The biggest problem was to get them together, and I felt the lack of a co-therapist. When I managed to get them both to come, the results were often dramatic. There is nothing new in this, but to me it was always a very satisfying experience. Sometimes it was too late, the relationship was past repair, as I had found in my own marriage. It coincided with the time when I was playing with the idea that most of us have more than one adolescence. In my own case the recent severance from the land of my fathers, the subsequent depression (the ice-age dream) and the fulfilment of childhood ambitions was, I thought, a good example. I could identify others as I reviewed my life.

A man in his late thirties came to see me. He had gone abroad as a young man where he had undergone a vasectomy, having become convinced, as some young people were at the height of the Cold War, that the world was going to be an unhealthy place in which to bring up children. He had now married, and both he and his wife regretted his earlier decision. They had of course been advised that, after so long, the chance of a successful reversal of the vasectomy was very small. My task was to help them to explore the situation, so that they could both reach a clear mode of thinking about their lives, uncluttered by doubts, 'if onlys' and recriminations. After many months of working together I had an intuitive feeling that an attempt should be made at reversal of the vasectomy. It was a feeling based on a sense that there would be something wrong with the natural order of things if this did not go right. Just a few times in my professional career I have had this feeling.

A year later this couple brought a healthy baby to the clinic. It was a beautiful and rewarding moment for all of us who had been involved in the case. John Guillebaud was looking for someone to take over vasectomy counselling, which I did shortly afterwards. In medicine it is difficult to avoid getting a one-sided view of society and of human nature. This clinic did much to redress that balance. There I saw whole families. It was a requirement that the patient brought his wife or partner, and I encouraged them to bring their children as well. There was much pleasure and reward in seeing so many dedicated, hard-working and cheerful families who felt their family was complete. At the session it was necessary to go into intimate discussion about anatomical and physiological matters. I found that the children would listen to what made sense to them, and turned off when it ceased to do so. It set me thinking that if sex education is to be taken seriously in our schools, the best way would be to involve the parents as well as the children in seminars on the subject.

My work in the psychosexual field brought into focus the subject which I can best categorise as 'Who should have children?'. The desire to mate, procreate and raise a family is probably the deepest-rooted of all archetypal constellations. The general loosening of social control and legal boundaries, together with the decline in religious practice, has deprived many young people of the essential psychological steps needed to become adult. Indeed, for many young women all they are left with to make them feel adult is to have a baby.

I know that to pose the question 'Who should have children?' has overtones of Huxley's *Brave New World* (1932) and the excesses of Nazi Germany. In the UK, as well as in other European countries, there was a strong movement during the 1920s and 1930s based on the idea that 'brains are better than brawn'. Indeed, Marie Stopes, in the course of her libel action in 1923, declared her social intentions in clear terms. She spoke of 'the steady evil which has been growing for a good many years of the reduction in the birth rate just on the part of the thrifty, wise, well-contented, and generally sound members of our community, and the reckless breeding from the C3 end, and the feeble-minded, the careless, who are proportionately increasing in our community because of the slowing of the birth rate at the other end of the social scale'. It is true that later in her evidence she declared what I believe to be true, that she was deeply concerned to improve the quality of life for poor and deprived families whose ignorance of birth control burdened them with far more children than they could manage. However, the eugenics issues is not my concern here, nor is it a debate that any longer has any life in it apart from a few extremists.

My real concern is the effect of the extension of the magic words 'the right to...' into almost every aspect of life. The influence of Freud and Jung in the first half of the 20th century appeared to have resulted in a rise in peoples' awareness that the real forces behind human wishes, behaviour and endeavour lie in the unconscious. In the second half this has become displaced by a growth of scientific and medical science. Indeed the technical discoveries in medicine have made it possible to smother or ignore age-old and deeply embedded archetypes. Today a woman may demand her 'absolute right' to have children at all costs. She may have children without the aid of a man, for the sperm to come from men who are not her husband; to have another woman carry her fertilised ovum; and to conceive and bear a child at any age over puberty. A woman whose husband is infertile would probably baulk at sleeping with another man in order to become pregnant. Nevertheless she is willing to accept the sperm from an unknown one. Accordingly, she must be doing violence to her unconscious. It will be the task of the psychotherapists of the 21st century to discover what effect this violation of the laws of the unconscious has, not only on the mother but also on the children born by the IVF programmes on offer and to come. It is no coincidence that the loosening of social boundaries, the loss of rites of passage and the absence of effective role models has been balanced by a great hunger among young people for new experiences, for alternative religions and lifestyles, and for mind-expanding drugs. It could be argued that this is a healthy development. It may suffice for a few years, but, in their thirties, women start to yearn for a child and men long for a more settled life where they once more matter in family life.

When I was working on these ideas, around the mid-1980s, I had several dreams which I identified as birth dreams. Their significance was that they took me into an archetypal place of mystery and legend. I dreamt of a cave which is used by many to reach a desired place. I walk across green meadows to this cave which I enter. From the cave I pass into a tunnel which could be dangerous, even fatal, to pass through. Eventually I come into the open air and find that I am close to the sea, where I meet a companion. The water is dark and surges back and forth with a rhythmic sound. Then I hear a baby crying softly, but there is no baby there. My companion says that this is a legendary place; that those who come to it always hear the cry of a baby. It is a moving and solemn moment, like that of the birth of a prince or the passing of a king.

In this dream I was in the land of birth. It is also the place of tension where the sea meets the land. Out of the sea came the life which populated the land. Creatures come out of the ocean to raise their young on the shore and then return to it. The cry of new life which I hear in the dream is a demand for creative action. Since the dawn of mankind women have interpreted the cry literally. It is too much to expect the 'liberated' Western woman of today to ignore it. There have always been women who turned their talents and their personalities into other fields. We cannot universally go back to 'traditional values', even though there are many families, perhaps more than we think, who have never abandoned them.

The dynamic psychologists of the 20th century taught that the real forces actuating human behaviour lie in the unconscious. They gave us more; they gave us an understanding of the nature of those forces. Jung, and to a lesser extent Freud, linked contemporary thought and behaviour to universal myths and legends going back to the beginning of recorded writing and story-telling. We cannot escape their force. It wells up and takes charge, sometimes when we least expect it. We define good and evil by whether it is appropriate to the moment or our situation or not. Orthodox Freudians speak of the harshness of the superego as determining our fate. This may be true for some. For me it is the superior power of unconscious forces threatening and overthrowing superego values which is a much more dangerous contribution to human instability and misery.

In the last chapter, I described my arrival in London in November 1982 and my attendance at the January workshop of the Group Analytic Society (London) in 1983. My experience there in Louis Zinkin's small group set me thinking once again about the question: 'What does constitute healing in the group?' It was an old question. In Southampton some of us had wrestled with it one summer when we got no further than putting the question. The chance came in 1987 when Adele Mittwoch and I convened the January workshop on the theme of healing agents in the group.

The kipper, illustrated, adorned the top of Adele's talk, as printed in *Group Analysis* (Mittwoch 1987), in which she began in Figure 6.1:

> Many of us here are in the business of getting patients better. We might ask ourselves what we mean by 'getting' and 'better'. I have used words that are

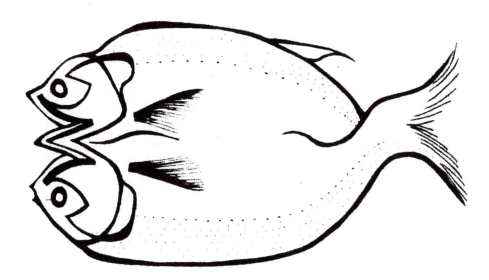

Figure 6.1 'Nothing is cured except a kipper' (from a drawing by Beth Sandison)

vague, undifferentiated, boundless. At the very beginning of this workshop I offer ideas that are basic, devoid of theory, undifferentiated.

I have heard it said that the only things that can be cured are kippers. I like a kipper for breakfast when grilled for me in a hotel in some lovely part of Scotland. The kipper starts off as a herring. It becomes a kipper through the process of curing, which in this case means the process of splitting open, cleaning, rubbing with salt and drying in woodsmoke. The effect of the curing is to alter the protein structure of the tissue. Curing in this sense is a process whereby something is being done to the fish to radically alter its structure. The herring, poor thing, is dead and presumably does not contribute, not even on an unconscious level.

The two verbs 'to heal' and 'to cure', according to the dictionaries I have consulted, are basically synonymous. (p.335)

My own paper (Sandison 1987) used a games metaphor on which the workshop might focus. Indeed, the theme of play as a healing force was strong throughout.

I want to develop four themes which I believe together constitute the healing potential of the small group (in doing so I assume that healing does take place in groups). I offer my views as to the agents which bring this about, which are (1) the nature of the group itself, (2) the conductor, (3) the setting, and (4) the process of initiation or 'getting-into' the group.

I start with an experience of my own which throws light on all four of these propositions. When I was about six years old and a stranger in the district to which we had just moved, I watched a group of children playing cricket on the green opposite our house. It was a fine warm summer evening but I was much too shy to join in. Then a neighbour came out and took me over to the group. Suddenly I was 'in', accepted, equal and with the hope of more good friendship next day. Indeed some of those kids remained my friends for several years.

Cricket is both similar to and different from a small group. Both, nevertheless, have well-defined boundaries but whereas cricket has precise rules, things in a group are much more open and flexible. However, the greatest reward in cricket, a six, comes from a stroke hitting the ball over the boundary, whereas the consequences of transgressing the boundaries in a small group may be embarrassing and uncomfortable. This metaphor from cricket leads me to the idea that there has to be a correspondence between inner and outer if therapy, either group or individual, is to be successful. In individual therapy meaning and healing are often only possible if there is or has been, current or past, a good relationship with someone, even if it means, as Winnicott (1971) reminds us, going back to our earliest infantile experience. Somewhere, sometime, therefore, we need to identify good group experiences 'out there' if we are to make sense of a small-group experience. Thus, I discovered as a six-year-old that acceptance and pleasure, which is part of living, arise simply from being in the group itself. (p.344)

From this, and from the great body of experience accumulated by group analysts, I conclude that just being in a small group has a healing potential.

I continued this theme with stories from games at Christmas parties, again of long ago in my childhood, and how one of my groups once took healing into its own hands by going outdoors and playing a game of 'twos and threes'.

This workshop confirmed my view that it is not 'treatment' which heals the patient – it is the quality of the relationship between therapist and patient. Playing a game with others establishes boundaries and cements or creates relationships, as I discovered long ago in my first game of cricket.

An enjoyable personal comment came from Barbara Robson (Robson 1987), which I must include, even if it is only to give myself a warm glow:

> Adele and Ronald, how I warmed to you, reassured by the respect and affection you clearly feel for each other, and heartened by your humour and compassion which seemed to shine through all you had to say. From this shared introduction our first shared image emerged. A delightful, and puzzling, symbol of the healing process. A glittering silver herring transformed by death, exposure and slow heat into something else, cured. A kipper! Bronzed, tasty, juicy, food. Better those with a backbone still intact, we agreed. Better than those spineless processed ones, Ichthus. The association moved me greatly, but I kept quiet, this time. (p.25)

This workshop was held in January 1987, four years after the one in which I had been in Louis Zinkin's group. Much had happened in my life. I commenced analysis with Louis in November 1984, and ended in July 1988. In the May before the workshop on healing I had a dream about being gradually sucked into the grinding routine of army life. I meet a group analyst, an old friend who invites me to join a group of good friends for a group analytic workshop. I do this, leaving a note for the commanding officer, but not without fantasies of being 'absent without leave', with men scouring the countryside for me. I was beginning to understand the nature of what I had been in thrall to for many years.

Beth and I were married in October 1986. It was a good occasion, attended by members of both our families. I recalled how none of my family had come to my 'wedding' of 1965. Beth and I had known each other for 18 years, but we nevertheless realised that we were taking a risk. Not long before we married I had a dream that we were newly wed. I saw her as awesomely beautiful, but then I realised that it was my first wife Evelyn that I was with, but she was also Beth. Thanks to the work that Louis and I did together, and to Beth's love and tolerance, we know that we belong. Our enduring fantasy is that we were washed up on the same beach. We recognised each other, and set off to make something of our good fortune.

On the night after the January workshop I dreamt that Beth and I were in Shetland, and that, on a beautiful starlit night, we go on a long journey by foot.

However, we get separated and I realise that it is the day of my mother's funeral. I feel a sad, indescribable sense of loss. Everyone had gone, and the undertaker and I bury my mother together.

I offer these dreams and thoughts without comment, except to say what will be clear to many, that an intensive small group workshop is always both healing and disturbing, throwing one back on unresolved, or partially resolved, psychic events.

The sense of loss continued to pursue me. I dream that Louis abandons me for a group. I dream also of astronomical events, mostly eclipses. In one dream the sun is not so much eclipsed as giving transit to a small object or moon across the sun. In another the sun is truly eclipsed, but each body is alternately light and dark.

For years I had been struggling to make sense of the most basic of all human conflicts, which is that between good and evil. The Group Analytic Society and Institute needed persuading that it was a valid theme. It is a common reaction. People think that this is a matter for theologians and churchmen to sort out and pronounce on. Unfortunately the Church tends to come up with the view that good is all right and evil is bad, which we knew anyway. The opportunity to express my own views on this matter came in February 1992, when the Institute held a two-day workshop on the subject.

Three years earlier I worked as a staff member at the January workshop entitled 'Envy and Jealousy'. It was convened by Gerald Wooster and Janet Boakes, and accordingly some innovations were to be expected. I particularly welcomed the 'entre acte', which took the form of story-telling; Billy Budd, Joseph and his brothers from the Book of Genesis, and a modern tale about an envious vicar. The convenors afterwards wrote (Wooster and Boakes 1989):

> We were on the whole a harmonious and co-operative team. We had one almighty row, but otherwise got on well. There were times when we thought that anxiety about envy between us was influencing how we behaved together.
>
> A suggestion which arose at the end was to have a consultant to the staff team. It would have been interesting and might have facilitated a deeper exploration of our own dynamics than we managed ... The committee have been vindicated in their choice of theme, but it also influenced staff relationships. (p.11)

The latter idea was adopted and at the next January workshop, I took on the role of consultant. It was a step forward on the path that the Society has been very reluctant to pursue, looking at its own dynamic. In fact it has never done so, and it is only now, looking back over the years, that I can see some of the issues more clearly. Envy and jealousy was a dynamic which troubled the Society for years. The committee exhibited an inverted envy by over-compensating for the envy or imagined envy of some of our European colleagues. At the same time there was an overvaluing of the supposed uniqueness of Foulkesian group analysis over all others. It has always seemed to me that the Group Analytic Society (London) should have developed as Foulkes himself wished it, as a London society with strong overseas connections. If others wished to learn about Foulkesian group analysis, they should come to London to do so. Enormous energy and efforts have been and are being expended by zealous members who conduct workshops abroad. It is exciting work, but I believe it tends to overlook the need of every culture to develop its institutions in its own way. It might have avoided a number of angry scenes at the Annual General Meeting, a sense of 'London cringe', and the formation of some breakaway groups who saw our efforts as missionary in nature.

This view is a personal one, and not very popular. Some of my best experiences overseas have been with diversity. The group analysts in Athens suffered grievous splits and in-fighting, but I found the workshop of the Institute of Group Analysis (Athens), which took place in Athens in April 1987, a most stimulating affair. The theme was working with psychotic patients in groups, and was one in which I have a special interest. The other workshops that I attended with pleasure were the 10th International Congress of Group Psychotherapy, Amsterdam, August 1989, and the 2nd Pacific Rim Congress in Group Psychotherapy, January 1991. The theme of the latter was 'Rapprochement', which reintroduced the concept of the healing process. I had gone, in part, because I wished to know how Australian colleagues go about their work, and I was not disappointed. There were 1200 participants in Amsterdam, from 32 countries. One of the aims of the congress was to construct it as a group experience in itself. The success of this was partly due to the emphasis on Moreno-style psychodrama, 'Playback Theatre' and 'Spontaneous Theatre', as well as the many reflective workshops and discussions. I left with a feeling that group psychotherapy and group analysis has much to offer at the level of conferences such as Amsterdam, and that too many missionary efforts may be divisive.

The workshop on 'Good and Evil' was held in February 1992. In Chapter 9, 'A Century of Psychotherapy', I describe my first encounter with the fact of good and evil at the age of ten. At the workshop Howard Cooper, a Rabbi and psychotherapist, spoke of the passage in the Book of Genesis in which Adam and Eve gained their knowledge of good and evil by eating the fruit of the tree of knowledge. He said: 'It would seem that this phrase...does not refer to sexual knowledge, or to moral and ethical knowledge, but to the human capacity to discriminate.' Unfortunately, in human society we find it hard to distinguish between 'sin' and evil, and this point was well taken in the workshop. My upbringing, from my earliest years, had been to do with learning that some things are good, like being polite to friends and relatives, while others are harmful, like the tops of hot stoves and overeating. When I read *The Robber Bridegroom* with such relish to my grandmother, good and evil were all one to me. After her reaction of disgust, I 'knew' the difference, and my knowing was a deeply archetypal affair.

It was refreshing to be able to realise that the God of the Old Testament was both good and bad. One of the problems for Christianity is that the Church has gradually split off all taint of darkness and evil from God. Satan was originally as much the 'bringer of light' as Christ himself. Christ, who is represented as free from all sin, nevertheless recognised the devil in himself during the temptations in the wilderness. The gospel writers externalised this evil into the person of Satan. Jung and Father Victor White struggled with this paradox and the problem that 'good' cannot exist by itself. White said it could and we should strive towards this greater good. Jung declared his fundamental opposition to this with the dictum 'the greater the good, the greater the evil'. Knowing that the Christian story had cast Satan out of heaven, he wondered whether he could ever be re-instated. If he were, it seems to me that at least we would know where he was, and our ability to discriminate between good and evil would be sharpened.

Questions of good and evil are not 'out there', they are relevant to the everyday work of the psychotherapist. We talked at the workshop about the old identification of depression with sin and evil. In the next section I will be talking about my special interest in the psychotherapy of depression. It was about the time of the 'Good and Evil' workshop that I had this dream:

> I am at home with Beth in the evening and we are relaxing. Answering a knock at the door I find a middle-aged woman accompanied by a black Labrador dog. She asks for an immediate consultation, which I agree to as she seems very distressed. She starts talking about her anxiety and her depression. While she is talking the black dog turns into a black snake. This snake fastens its jaws on my left shoulder and holds on while she continues to unburden herself. At length she finishes and the snake relaxes its hold. Then she says, 'I feel much better now, and I will leave the snake with you.' She leaves, but I do not see the black snake again. Instead there is a black cat curled up on the doormat.

The black cat contains both good and evil, he is the bringer of good fortune and the familiar of witches. Discrimination here is uncertain. We encourage our patients to 'unburden themselves'. It is important in the practice of psychotherapy to look rather carefully sometimes at what they do leave. It is not always 'rubbish'.

CHAPTER 7

3. Individual Psychotherapy, Psychotherapy and Depression, Context and Place. LONDON 1982–1992

The four facets of my professional life described in these three chapters headed 'London' feel today like elements having an equal emotional value. But individual psychotherapy occupied the bulk of my time. The practice of psychotherapy has been a ruling principle in my life for over 50 years. When I was thinking about this I asked myself where and how did the psychotherapist in me have its (or his or her) origins. Fortunately, a dream came to my aid at the crucial moment.

I dreamt that I was in a large farmhouse. It was evening. There were going to be many people for breakfast, and my task was to prepare the meal. I went to bed and had a dream that shifted from inner to outer. I was getting this meal together, and then I was exploring the unconscious, moving into outer space, or perhaps inner space, where it was dark blue. There I saw the archetypes of the collective unconscious, truly nebulous and difficult to focus on. Then they would become clearer and look like spiral nebulae – galaxies in the heavens.

I saw a middle-aged woman lying on a bed. An analyst appeared, perhaps Jung himself, who said, 'She will never make a success of her marriage, she cannot reach the unconscious.'

It was early the next morning, and I got up to prepare, single-handed, this breakfast feast. I found a long trestle table, laid for about 20 people. One of my grand-daughters was busy at it. She was an amalgam of all four of my elder son's daughters. She knew that this was a feast to celebrate the archetypes. Not everyone could partake. She brought in quantities of food, large joints of beef, cereals, bread, dairy products, eggs, all from the farm. One of my grand-daughters had to leave, and she took her two children and went out through the back door.

I walked along a wide corridor, and opened a door which led to a beach. It was sandy and divided into two parts by a skerry, although one could get from one side to the other. On the far beach was a great boulder, oval in shape, and pinkish, like a Shetland boulder from Northmavine. The sea was very rough, with big breakers on the shore. One of these rolled this huge boulder up and round to the near beach. It could be dangerous. The power of the ocean was enormous. After it came to rest I opened the door and went back into the wide corridor.

In this dream I was using the image of a nebula, a galaxy outside our own, as an image to understand the nature of the archetypes of the collective unconscious. I was moving from inner to outer – that is, from my way of imagining it to pictures of the collective from my unconscious, my dreaming self. One cannot actually 'see' an archetype, and those nebulae came and went in my dream. They took me back to those wonderful, magical days of discovery, long ago, when astronomy was my ruling passion. Figure 7.1 is from *The Universe Around Us*, by James Jeans (1929). I was 13 years old when I read this book.

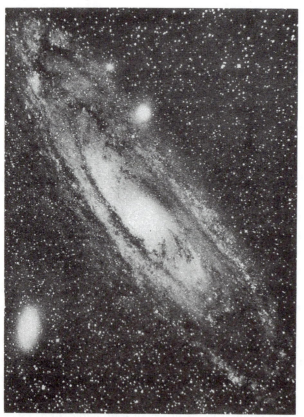

Figure 7.1 The Great Nebula (M31) in Andromeda. The spiral nebula illustrates my dream of the collective unconscious.

In my 13-year-old mind deep questions arose. Why is the universe there? What does it mean? Surely there must be other life there, somewhere. If the universe had a beginning, as Jeans said, what came before the beginning? Jeans spoke of the beginning being like 'the finger of God stirring the ether'. So God must have been there before the beginning. No one in my childhood had an answer to these riddles. Seventy years later, we are not much further along that road, but it is now clearer to me why they remain mysteries.

I could expand upon my need to explore, to look at first causes and first principles and to experience rather than unravel mystery. My choice of the Royal Air Force during the war, and abandoning medicine for the physiology of breathing and seeing, may have had their roots in the telescope and laboratory of my earlier days. My life has been one of many changes in a world that has changed almost beyond recognition, and so it is comforting to seek a unifying principle. The words which inspired me to study Jung and all his works in 1947 were those like 'anima', 'mandala' and 'archetype'. And here they are again, in a dream more than 50 years later. The difference is that, what was a seductive invitation long ago is now an integral part of my way of looking at people and things. I can understand how my four grand-daughters became a kind of group anima. Last summer Lucy and I had long talks about our experiences of a sense of place. I had written a very personal essay about this which I had intended, one day, to give my sons. But I gave it to her. In the sunshine we sat on a grassy bank overlooking the river valley, and she told me about a powerful and symbolic dream she had had when she was a child. We had done that rare thing, meeting consciously at an unconscious level. I have had similar experiences with Ali and Gemma, but they were not so far developed. Perhaps one day I could have a similar relationship with the fourth grand-daughter who left the house, but she has taken a different path and is lost to me at the moment. As the dream said, she left by the back door.

When I recall my patients, and look again at the notes I wrote, and at the letters I have written, I know that the practical business of therapy is different. One does not always enter the deep recesses of the collective unconscious, or watch the anima guide one's patient into self-discovery. Psychotherapy is mostly about the relationship between two people, the fact of just being together and working on problems, hang-ups and the clash of opposites, or whatever. Nevertheless, analysts of whatever school ignore the manifestations of the unconscious at this deep level at their peril. A choice has to be made, as Jung is believed to have discovered, or, as he would have said, was fated to make. His most recent biographer, Hayman (1999), reports that after his fiftieth birthday he tried hard to cut down on his patients and to devote more time to scientific writing and work. He was said to have been permanently ambivalent towards his patients. The length of analysis with most was much shorter than is customary today, and his habit of sharing his dreams and personal ideas and fantasies with his patients would be considered very unorthodox today. Several of his earlier patients became competent and distinguished analysts. His wife Emma was also drawn into the magic circle. In the early days of analysis its pioneers needed to create a family of therapists.

I can recall one or two of my patients who have successfully trained as therapists. It is hard to be sure of the part which transference dynamics played in this. Another started training at medical school, which did seem to be the result of some unresolved transference and counter-transference issues. However, he gave it up during the second year, which was probably appropriate. I have come across some patients who patently needed a complete change of direction in their lives, and many achieved just that. The commonest career result of psychotherapy has been advancement and promotion in the patient's chosen field. I am sure that this reflects some less conscious quality in myself. It is even tempting to speculate that the patients benefited at my expense. I comfort myself that our family has never been adept at amassing a fortune.

The theme of loss and its close relative, depression, has occupied me for many years. During the 20th century volumes were written on the clinical aspects of it, adopting the medical model which translates depression into an illness. Most of the names connected with it, such as Kraepelin, Adolf Meyer, Eugen Bleuler, Winakur and others, did an immense amount of research and presumably a lot of thinking. They have left us with a few rather unsatisfactory concepts about depression, without adding much to our understanding of its nature.

Both Freud and Jung linked depression with the inescapable fact of death. Freud's paper on *Mourning and Melancholy* was published in 1917 (Freud 1924–1950). Jung wrote his celebrated *Answer to Job* in 1952 (Jung 1958). He says in the preface that he had been concerned with the central problem posed by Job for years. His long correspondence with the English Dominican priest Victor White very probably had a lot to do with his decision to write at length on the subject. Jung reminds us that the Old Testament God 'knew no moderation of his emotions and suffered precisely from this lack of moderation. He himself admitted that he was eaten up with rage and jealousy and that this knowledge was painful to him (p.365)'. Jung says that his concern was 'the way in which a modern man with a Christian education and background comes to terms with the divine darkness which is unveiled in the book of Job, and what effect it has on him' (p.365). Jung viewed the story of Job as one step in the development of human consciousness. He brings the proposition into the 20th century. Very briefly, Christ and the Apocalypse separated the God of the Trinity, who was all good, from Satan, who carried all the evil. But it was made clear that man carried both good and evil and was responsible for the consequences. Jung says: 'He can no longer wriggle out of it on the plea of his littleness and nothingness, for the dark God has slipped the atom bomb and chemical weapons into his hands and given him the power to empty out the apocalyptic vials of wrath on his fellow creatures' (p.461).

Depression, melancholy, lowering of spirit and despair are ways of describing something we are all familiar with at some time in our lives. It always has been so, it is part of the human condition. The concept of melancholy has permeated literature from earliest times. Scholars and divines from Aristotle onwards have tried to explain and describe melancholy from the standpoint of their age, but always leaned towards rationalism. The great 16th century work of Robert Burton, *The Anatomy of Melancholy* (1927 Edition), must be read in this context. Much of this huge book is devoted to melancholy as a human condition – for example, when he writes about love-sickness. Although he has been seen as 'a scholarly and humanistic precursor of Freud' (Dell and Jordan-Smith, eds, 1927, p.xiii), Burton relied on the authority of earlier physicians, Galen, Hippocrates, Avicenna and others. He could not make up his mind about depression. Sometimes he blames God, at others, man's own folly, sometimes it is a pure human condition, at others an illness, amenable to medical treatment with Borage or Hellebore. He even wrote of 'the sweet joy of melancholy', but few in its grip would agree today.

Twentieth century doctors have tried to simplify and unify melancholy by making it into an illness, an abnormal and pathological state. Worse, they have proposed heroic methods of 'treatment' which to many seem as primitive and barbarous as the ducking stool and the whirling centrifuges of earlier times. We now have had a galaxy of medicaments, prescribed with such freedom as to give the impression that the whole world is depressed. And perhaps it is. I recall Carl Meier's statement to me in 1952, quoted in Chapter 2, that, since the war, the English had lost their soul. At about the same time Arthur Bryant (1953) made a similar remark about the Anglo-Saxons of the first millennium AD. He believed that they had become afflicted with hopelessness, 'behind their cold inexorable heavens lay only terror and disaster' (p.14). Much the same sentiment could be applied to our society today. The media, especially radio and television, which can invade the privacy of our homes 24 hours a day, feed us with a constant stream of disasters, stories of disability, anguish, despair and death, culled from every corner of the globe. This would not happen if the readers, listeners and viewers were not emotionally tuned and ready to identify with this input. Perhaps, in a macabre way, Burton was right after all when he spoke of the 'sweet joy of melancholy'.

In 1963, supported by the clergy group, I was instrumental in starting the Worcester branch of the Samaritans. In subsequent years I gave several talks to 'Nightline', a student organisation set up at a number of universities as a telephone helpline for students with depression or suicidal ideas. One of these, given in Southampton, was published in *The Lancet* (R.A. Sandison 1972). It was written during a very depressed and unsettled phase in my own life during which I recorded no dreams or personal experiences. I was preoccupied with the idea that depression is either a sin or the result of sin. 'Sin' was defined as 'lack of faith, moral fibre or social responsibility' (p.1227). I argued that by labelling the condition as 'depressive illness' the sufferer avoids punishment and is treated tolerantly and in a way which creates dependency and trust. I comment that 'this has certain advantages' (p.1227). I went on to say that depressives are often looking for punishment and recognition, citing the case of shoplifting in a depressed middle-aged woman. The Act repealing suicide as a criminal act dated from 1963, only nine years earlier, and people had been imprisoned for attempting suicide as late as 1960. At that time a consultant physician told me that he could scarcely bear to treat attempted suicides in his wards as he was convinced that they had brought the condition on themselves. Even today one hears about suicides in which even close members of the family appeared to have no knowledge that the person was depressed.

My view in 1972, and since then, has been that although a certain number of people with depression are 'ill' in the medical sense, we would do better in most cases to see depression as a natural although painful condition of man, and its intensification as a product of our age and social culture. The outward manifestation of depression in society is violence, and violent acts and crime tend to proceed from those whose social deprivation, poverty of spirit and lack of constructive goals have dragged them into depression and despair.

From the 1960s until the present day, many of my patients in psychotherapy have been depressives. There is a myth that depressive patients are inaccessible to therapy. In my paper I noted a study carried out in Portsmouth (Barraclough et al. 1970) on one hundred people who had committed suicide. Forty per cent had sought professional help within a week of their death, and 60 per cent within a month. The depression had entered a phase whereby the patient ceased to project his problems on to others and consequently had become a problem to himself. This is the point of self-revelation. The sad thing is that he or she is often not heard, being offered a prescription for antidepressants and sent away. When the patient subsequently kills himself it is revealed that he sought medical help, for which he was 'treated', so no blame attaches to anyone.

It is not my purpose to write a treatise on depression in this book. I have had the privilege of spending many therapeutic hours with patients who have either contemplated suicide or attempted it, and I have witnessed their relief at being heard at last, and had the reward of observing the depression lifting. There is another category for people who may ruminate about suicide, but who seldom or never do so. This state has been described as non-being, and was well described by Paul Tillich (1952). I wrote at the time that the sufferers were often young, and that 'these are not those whom the gods love, and are thus destined to die young, they are those whom the gods appear to have abandoned' (p.1228). These are indeed difficult people to help, but I have tried to adapt a Jungian dictum, which can be formulated as 'the greater the deprivation and loss, the greater the need for love'. It is a dangerous area of transference and counter-transference for the therapist, and many do not care to embark on it.

Indeed, there are some psychoanalysts who cannot work with depressives. I was surprised and gratified at the large number of letters I received in response to my paper. They were all very positive except one which came from a Danish psychoanalyst with whom I had worked earlier, during the 'LSD period' (see Chapter 2). Dr Vanggaard wrote me a very angry letter, saying: 'How *could* you serve up to us all this Laingish stuff, even applied to depression of all conditions?' He and a colleague sent a letter to *The Lancet* advocating that depressives should be treated with anti-depressants, electro-convulsive treatment or 'prevented by lithium salts'. It was and is a view held by many. However, that it should be held by an analyst was astonishing. It led me, of course, to reflect on the intense reaction of jealousy which my international reputation in the field of LSD therapy had aroused a few years earlier, and which was still rumbling on. I am not sure whether *The Lancet* ever published that letter, as I have no record of it. Anyway, I may never know the whole story, as at the same time I received a letter from another Danish analyst who thanked me for 'your dignified and valuable presentation of depression'. Another, which I value, came from a biochemist in Leiden, Holland, who referred to Sylvia Plath's book *The Bell Jar (1998),* which he had read. 'It is a good description of the "not being" state of a young person, a gifted American writer who eventually committed suicide. Since she describes her treatment so accurately one also wonders if she could have been saved if psychotherapy had taken the place of ECT.' I had ventured to throw some light on human emotions, so I should not have been surprised to have an intensely emotional response. I believed passionately in what I had written. The angry rebuff from Vanggaard took me right back to the vulnerability of childhood, when an unguarded remark to parents or teachers can trigger a response which makes one feel like an outcast.

To this I add a footnote. It has been my experience, and that of other analysts with whom I have discussed the matter, that suicide during the course of therapy is very unusual. We know that those who live alone or have nobody who matters to them are most at risk. A good therapeutic relationship is a vital bridge to the alienated and despairing. It is a bridge towards more lasting relationships when therapy ends. I had worked with a patient for two years or more when she went through a long period of self-destructive despair. One afternoon in early spring she left my consulting room. Travelling home on the bus she decided to kill herself. She had the necessary pills all ready when she got home. The sun was setting and she wrote a note saying goodbye, not to people, but to nature. Then she thought about her therapy, and how she would never see me again, and a warm desire for her next session overcame her despair. She came and told me all this a few days later. This account may sound dramatic, life and death are serious matters, but I am convinced to this day that, but for the transference, I would not have seen her again.

There are those whose suicide seems appropriate from the outside. We can never fully understand the minds of those whom we do not know intimately. There is much scope and need for therapy for some people with terminal illness, particularly cancer. I have almost no experience of this. I do take the view that the saving or prolongation of life at all costs is out of step with the order of things.

Some who read this may ask what I offer my patients, and how I go about my work. The answer is that I have no set way, and I cannot easily describe what I do in words. I might glibly say that the only way to find out would be to come and present yourself as a patient. If you have read this far I hope you will have got some idea, because I have given a context to my professional life. You will certainly have learned far more about my life than I ever reveal to a patient. However, therapists work in consulting rooms which usually say a great deal about them. I am no exception, and much of my history is locked up in coded form among the contents of my room. That is the difference. You, the reader, have the words, and some of the facts. The way I work therapeutically is coded within those words. The patient experiences our interaction, while my personality and history lie coded within the room. This is not a teasing riddle, it is a fact of life.

When in London I gave an annual lecture in Northampton entitled 'The Context of the Group'. Its purpose was to illustrate connections between group setting and group behaviour and experience. Much the same exercise could be applied to individual therapy. The archetypal group, say a palaver or a group round a camp fire, meets in the open. Freud and Jung, and no doubt other early analysts, often went for long walks with their patients, and these were claimed to have been therapeutic. There is more sense in groups being in the open when the place of meeting is the same each time and thus forms the context. On a long walk the points of reference are always changing. Perhaps for this reason, analysts have now retreated with their patients behind firmly closed doors, often double to ensure soundproofing. No telephone rings, no interruptions are permitted. However, there has to be a clock. Some have likened this room with its constant environment to the womb, and the ticking of the clock to the maternal heart beat. This is not my fantasy. I see my consulting room as the place where my patient and I have each other's full attention for the duration of the analytic hour. Within that the patient can go anywhere in words and imagination. There is no set agenda. The romance and excitement of the hour is that at its beginning we never know where we will be at its end. Sometimes a patient comes saying that he has nothing to say. Fifty minutes later it is hard to end the session.

From the beginning we commence a journey together, my patient and I. It is not a journey limited to the analytic hour. Patients have told me that in between sessions they have conversed with me, and put questions to me in fantasy. And we are not alone in the consulting room. Often it is peopled with the patient's family. Indeed, troublesome parents are sometimes hard to get rid of so as to leave us some privacy. This goes for me also. If I find myself drawn into parental injunctions with my patient I usually tell him so.

Place and events are inextricably linked. In 1975, when I left the house near Southampton, I sat in the almost empty consulting room for a long time. I thought of all that had happened in that room. It still carried an aura of the many histories, confessions, cries of anguish and fear. I thought also of some of the joys of discovery that had occurred. I reflected on the patient hours spent working towards a hoped-for goal. It was a room empty of all but memories.

I have often experienced beauty of place and human suffering as opposites. When they clash it causes me discomfort, even unbelief. I recall gazing with a kind of shock at a boatload of children arriving in Interlaken one golden summer's afternoon destined for a child guidance clinic, as if no pain should be allowed to disturb the beauty of the setting. One gets taken unawares by such primitive notions in unguarded moments.

It is part of the human condition to link crucial and emotional events with place. It is the syndrome enshrined in, 'Where were you when you heard that Kennedy had been shot?' This icon has been so overworked that its power and significance may have been lost. We should not talk about such matters. My experiences of where I was at times of great importance and significance have meaning only to me. They are likely to bore other people. Nevertheless, the psychic situations of our patients are always connected with the particular concerns and meaning of the time. Years ago a patient told me that when the Second World War broke out it also broke out in her head. Indeed the fortunes and disasters of that war reverberated among my patients for the remainder of the century, and may well spill over into the 21st. For some reason I have found myself involved with those whom the war displaced from Poland more often than might be ascribed to chance. I have been pursued by the guilty knowledge that while we were fighting for our survival in 1940 we overlooked the fact that we had originally declared war with the intention of liberating Poland from the iron grip of Nazism. In 1942, I started working with night fighter squadrons in training with the object of teaching them about the physiology of night vision and the use of oxygen. By chance, if there is indeed such a thing, the trainee aircrews at this station were nearly all Poles who had somehow found their way to this country. Each one had a tragic history, but I rarely got to know what it was. So much was lost in translation.

After the war, at Warlingham, I met Dr Ruth Hoffman, also a refugee from Poland, whose linguistic skills came to my aid. It was she who translated Stoll's account of Albert Hofmann's earliest work in Basel with LSD. Without that I might have hesitated to proceed as I did. Over the years we became close; there was always an unspoken bond between us, perhaps to do with our joint northern ancestry. More, we were both exiles although we shared very little about our personal lives. Then I worked for a long time with a Polish patient whose whole family had been annihilated in the gas chambers, to which, at the age of 13, she had been a witness. She was Jewish, although the majority of the Poles I knew and worked with were Catholics. Many Jews living in Poland identified themselves not as Polish, but as Jews living in Poland. They had a double sense of alienation.

Through the years I had other Polish patients, and I worked for several years with such a lady while I was in London. She had memories of the place she had known as a child, but had never been back. While in therapy she had a strong urge to return, full as she was of memories of the street where her grandparents had lived. She discovered that the town had been completely destroyed during the war, and that no trace of where they had once lived could be found. This actual total annihilation of the physical signs of her past was beyond my experience. However, living through this with her helped me to clarify some of the feelings I had had when I returned to Shetland to work in 1975. I had hoped I would feel I belonged and would be welcomed as a returning exile. Instead I had the feeling that I was a wanderer in a country which I had once known but which had changed beyond recall or recognition.

My father's youngest sister spent the war years nursing in Scotland where she formed a special attachment to the many Polish servicemen she had nursed. She had lost her only son at the hands of the Japanese in 1943. As a powerful compensation she made her patients into her sons, and she kept up correspondence with many until she died in 1981. While I was in Shetland I visited her in Sutherland as often as I could, where she lived alone after my uncle died. I have always thought of her as the psychotherapist of her generation in the family. She was rather crippled in her old age, and many visited her to tell their troubles. They always received affection and comfort, but she seldom advised. Children loved her and there seemed always to be two or three in the house. I loved her too, and she would tell me stories about a way of life in Shetland which she grew up with, and of which now only traces and substitutes remain. I understood how she identified so strongly with her Polish 'sons'.

They also called her their mother. After my Aunt Emily died I wrote to as many as possible. Some had settled in this country, several had returned to Poland. Ernest Piecha, writing from Rybnik, wrote: 'I got your letter with real sadness. My mummy has died. I will remember her in my thoughts and in my prayers ... I knew them in Lairg. In 1947 I left Lairg forever but we remained in conversation and we knew from each other what was to be known.' All the letters were addressed to 'My Dear Mummy', or 'Dearest Mammy'. Much may be 'lost in translation' but the manner in which Ernest described his relationship with a woman he would never see again needs no amendment: 'We remained in conversation and we knew from each other what had to be known.' My heart went out to these men with long memories. Analysts reading this will be tempted to see Emily as an enslaving mother who could not let her sons go. This is to devalue mothering at its best. I am personally sensitive to the seductions of the devouring mother, and I never felt it with her.

Eva Hoffman left Poland with her family in 1958 to live in Canada. She was 13 years old. She wrote (Hoffman 1997): 'And by what quirk of history, I wonder, has it come about that from the age of thirteen on I have not known what peace of mind feels like, that it strikes me as a phrase from another world. Is it that I come from the war, while my parents were born before it?' (p.129) There is no answer to this and the author wisely does not attempt it.

I commenced this chapter with a dream about the embedding of archetypes in our family psyche. I see a card opposite me as I write which I received last Christmas from the Polish patient mentioned above. One of the consequences of her depression had been a loss of the will and the ability to paint. She reminds me of her success in regaining the muse by sending a card each year which she has illustrated. The one I am looking at has on it a circular drawing depicting the conjunction of the sun and the moon. It could almost have come from an alchemical mediaeval treatise, but I know that it came from her. She wrote that she is having an exhibition of her work at a major festival this year. During four years in therapy we struggled to find her creativity, and I would annoy her by always being hopeful about this. She found it herself, and has sustained it through the nine years since. Her drawing arrived at a powerful season when the inexorable march of time closed the 20th century and the second millennium and took us into the unknown of the third. Last year there was a total eclipse of the sun, this year there has been a total eclipse of the moon. Such events draw our attention to the opposites. In the one the moon obscures the sun, in the other the shadow of the earth obscures the moon. The sun disappeared completely for a short time, but the moon remained mysterious and coppery in colour. Perhaps the power of the feminine can never be lost, because it is cloaked in filmy mystery.

I was 11 years old when the only other total eclipse of the sun to be visible in this country in the 20th century took place. Of the first I saw nothing, as cloud covered the sun. There was only a darkening of the sky on a June morning and the birds stopped singing for a time. I saw the beginning of the second, and then clouds covered it. I was drawn to the first through science into mystery, to the second by mystery as much as science, coupled to a sense of *déjà vu*. I was at first tempted to think of the two eclipses as beginnings and endings, but they were neither. They were markers. At age 11 my unconscious was quietly allowing me to know who I was. Seventy-two years later I am more conscious of its archetypal power. My dreams since I started writing this chapter have warned me, once again, that it is not to be trifled with.

CHAPTER 8

Reflections

In the last chapter I wrote about some of my psychotherapeutic journeys with my patients during the 'London ten years', 1982–1992. Inevitably material from earlier periods crept in. I am conscious that almost every chapter has ended with loss and mourning, only to be followed in the next by some new adventure in my life. The unifying principle has been individual and group psychotherapy. I hope I have given some idea of the nature both of myself and of some of my patients. The current discussion about the value of psychotherapy favours the quality of the relationship between the two people over the brand of therapy they subscribe to. The problem is that we never get to hear much about the therapist. Therapists write about what they do rather than about who they are.

In previous chapters I have tried to give some idea about how the therapist in me grew. I try now to take a broader look at this process and how it has shaped my idea of how psychotherapy, psychoanalysis and its derivatives can be judged on the scale of human endeavour.

In 1991 I was 75 years old. The National Health Service had rather belatedly discovered that I was a bit past their retiring age, and I left the Margaret Pyke Centre at the end of that year. I said goodbye at its annual Christmas dinner at the Piccadilly Hotel. I left with feelings of great affection and regret. Regret not only about my severance from a place and people whom I had loved, but for the passing of an era. The clinic in Soho Square was probably one of the last which I recognised as having the same spirit of comradeship and adventure with which I was so familiar at King's before the war. Quite soon after I left, some of its key people retired, and it moved. It could never be the same again.

Beth and I had been exploring places in which to live outside London for a while. One Saturday afternoon in February 1992 we found ourselves in this town, and walked into the nearest estate agent on an impulse. In June we moved in. It is a move we have never regretted. I continued practising in London until November, as I wanted to give my patients good endings to therapy. I had planned to continue until the end of the year, but a spell of ill-health ordained differently. Ledbury is romantically described as the place of cider, hops and poets. Some of the poets get mention in the next and final chapter, but it may not be out of place to say that the poet laureate John Masefield's centenary falls this year, and that he was born in this town. Ledbury has also the romance and the history associated with border country and the Welsh Marches. Once more I find myself in the land between two cultures. How else could I escape this life-long fate, having a Shetland father and an English mother, and shuttling between the two cultures all my life? The years I have lived here have allowed me to grow and reflect on this and many things. I conclude that I need this tension in my life to fuel the creative aspects of my nature. Among other matters, I have been able to reflect on how I got to this point in my life. And now I return to my salad days in learning about psychotherapy.

In the autumn of 1934, during the term in which I started the study of anatomy, physiology and pharmacology, my attention was drawn to a lecture course in psychoanalysis by J.A. Hadfield. Two lectures a week for the winter terms over two years were on offer, so I signed up. Human anatomy is about *dissection*, the taking apart of the dead body to discover its component parts and the relations between them. Physiology was different. The hidden functions of the living body were explored and exposed. What Dr Hadfield offered was a context for the anatomy and physiology which I was about to study. There were precursors to my action. Out driving with my mother at the age of eight we would sometimes pass the great LCC asylums at Epsom and see crocodiles of patients going for an afternoon walk. My mother would comment on their look of 'queer-ness', and talk of heredity... Who were these people, and wasn't I lucky not to be one of them? And four or five years later she fell into a severe depression and our family life fell apart. She didn't look 'queer' as she lay languidly in the afternoons on a couch in the drawing room. I thought she looked rather lovely; a kind of serene beauty, held in suspension. But she had no desire to do anything and feared to go out of the house. One day when I was 16 I came home from school and she was still the same, and I said simply, 'When are you going to get better?'

Fifty years later, when she was in her nineties, and while talking to her, she told me that those words had come as a revelation. It was the point at which her recovery began, and she never fell into that dark pit of depression again. I have never forgotten J.A. Hadfield and his many stories about his patients, and how together they unravelled the psychopathology of the symptoms which they brought. His practice was not dominated by adherence to any one 'school' of analysis. He used them all as appropriate, and was very aware of the diverse needs of people of different ages and of varying backgrounds and interests. He was a religious man and had analysed a number of clergy. This perhaps was another facet of him which I resonated with and carried with me until, years later, I was able to make use of it in my own practice. His book (Hadfield 1936) is now probably forgotten. What I have not forgotten is the way he presented his material and the precision of his time-keeping. His demonstration of self-discipline set something in motion in my inner self which I came to value increasingly.

Dr Hadfield had given me permission to exercise discipline and patience. Felix was a young man, not much older than I, and he lay in the surgical ward at King's following surgery for Crohn's disease. His wound had become septic and liberally exuded pus which was dressed daily. I was his surgical dresser, and for nigh on six months I dressed his wound every day. It was a slow and painful procedure which took about an hour. In 1938 we had no sulphonamides, no antibiotics. We relied on the crude antiseptic power of mercurials and other organic chemicals. He and I would talk. I know we talked, but he told me very little about himself, and I hesitated to talk about my busy and active life because I realised that he would probably never enjoy such pleasures. What we shared most was our mutual patience. I somehow never thought that he would die. But one morning I walked into the ward and saw that his bed was empty. At that moment the house surgeon appeared. He was a good doctor and a Christian man. He said simply: 'I think it was best, one hundred units of insulin and four grains of morphia, that's all.' One could make that kind of decision in the days when life was more pragmatic, and issues of life and death were clearer, if they ever were. Felix and I had both been delivered from a long and painful event by the twin disciplines of hospital practice and my own persistence. I have never forgotten him, whose great black eyes stared mutely at me as I approached his bed each morning, noting as I did the unchanging nature of his temperature chart of 'hectic' fever, and seeing his face gradually shrink around his questioning, searching eyes. I learned so much from him – above all, I learned that I possessed patience. He taught me how and when to use it.

Recently I was discussing with Malcolm Pines how I came into psychiatry. He assumed that I had been involved with the subject in the Services during the war, as so many of my contemporaries were. However, it was physiology which had claimed my interest, as my first degree was in that subject. It came about as a result of a chance conversation. How many changes in my life have had their origin in a so-called chance encounter! I had joined the Royal Air Force Volunteer Reserve in 1941, without a clear idea as to where it would take me, but my thoughts were on flying and working as a squadron medical officer. I found myself posted to a medical board, examining a constant stream of air-crew volunteers. It served for a few months while I got used to service ways, and my colleagues on the Board were agreeable. The station in Bedfordshire was something of a transit zone for innumerable officers who came and went on missions varying from the humdrum to the top secret. One evening I got talking with one of them over a drink or two, which lasted far into the night. He was a doctor in a state of high arousal. His fiancée had recently been killed in an air-raid on London, and he was full of fire, passion and anger. 'Get out of here at all costs, get into the action, do everything you can!' was the thrust of his message. The effect on me was overwhelming. I have wondered since whether there is such a thing as a chance meeting; in retrospect it feels as if I was unconsciously waiting for the moment, and that everything subsequent to that was planned and orderly.

I wrote the next day and within a week I was posted to the Royal Air Force physiological laboratory at Farnborough, which in 1944 became the RAF Institute of Aviation Medicine. There, to my pleasure, I met the cream of the Cambridge physiologists. The team was headed by Bryan Matthews, a most likeable and friendly man. He was dedicated to the problems faced by aircrew, lack of oxygen, decompression sickness and the effects of positive and negative acceleration, 'G'. He seldom talked about himself, but I learned that he, like John Scott Haldane, had studied the effects of high altitude in the Andes in the 1930s. On that first visit I also met Professor Winfield, who pioneered the polar air routes after the war, Lamplough and others. Squadron Leader Bill Stewart, a fearless investigator and intrepid aviator, was working on high-altitude problems and on the effects of positive and negative 'G' on pilots. Bill Goldie, from University College, London, was researching the visual problems of night flying, a subject which occupied much of my time later on. He worked with a dedication and passion which only war can sustain, and his early death, from cancer of the lung, before its end was a great sadness.

My work, which was mostly in the field, took me to many places, and from it I cherish many memories and stories. It demanded the creation of training programmes in the twin areas of breathing and sight. The aircraft of the Second World War were unpressurised, but were nevertheless capable of reaching altitudes and speeds about which their effects on the body relatively little was known. I had the privilege of teaching pilots in the final stage of their operational training some of the paradoxical effects of high altitude and how this could be combated. I was glad that I had studied John Scott Haldane's meticulous work on altitude when, like Matthews, he conducted experiments at 17,000 to 18,000 feet in the Andes, and I remembered how the Mount Everest expeditions had captured my imagination as a boy. At that age I had spent many hours in the true darkness of our garden with my small telescope studying and recording astronomical objects. There I learned about dark adaptation, peripheral vision at night and how to scan the sky. Those evening hours in the winter demanded patience, and patience again came to my aid as I tried to convey knowledge of self-preservation to young men whose whole instinct was to disregard safety and get at the enemy. I had to devise means of demonstrating and convincing pilots that, in the process of ascending to 30,000 feet in a Spitfire in six minutes, a stage of pleasant euphoria is reached on the way unless oxygen is turned on early. It was that euphoria which sadly resulted in too many pilots losing consciousness and spinning to their deaths in the early days. It can still happen today if a modern aircraft loses cabin pressure.

There was something more. I found myself at the forefront of knowledge and technology in this particular field. It had the same effect on me as listening to my physics master at school describe Lindemann's experiments with atomic fission, hearing the Supermarine aircraft breaking records on Southampton water, seeing the million-volt 'lightning' discharge at the National Physical Laboratory, or watching the beating of the isolated perfused rabbit's heart. Later, it carried me into developing LSD as a therapeutic tool, and with any activity which carried me into new territory. It is a dangerous place to be, inflation and exploitation of the new territory can readily occur. It has happened to many, perhaps because they stayed too long in one field.

In those war years I taught night fighter pilots about the subtleties of night vision. I had models made and we set up demonstrations in dark rooms and decompression chambers. I owed much to Bill Goldie, who made me a beautiful photometer, with a finely balanced Wheatstone bridge which enabled me to reproduce night illumination from starlight to bright moonlight. All this I set up in what became known as the Night Vision Training Centre at High Ercall in Shropshire. This training culminated in what was to be the most hectic six weeks of my life. I set out on 12 April 1944 and visited every night fighter squadron in the country that was assembling for the D-Day assault on occupied Europe. I pay tribute to the discipline and dedication of their squadron commanders who invariably collected their crews together for my talk and demonstration which lasted about an hour. I always tried to mingle with them at night in their dispersal areas. There is something about the intimacy of the nights in Southern England in spring time which came to my aid. I was not so much concerned about making them more efficient fighting men, but I hope to this day that what I did helped a few to survive the war who might otherwise never have returned.

There are, of course, many more stories from those astonishing times. These few paragraphs alone must serve to describe one of the many transitional phases of my life, this time from the amateur astronomer and student of physiology to a teacher combining both disciplines. Breathing and seeing are two powerful metaphors which we constantly use in psychotherapy. We speak of the dark night of the soul, of 'light dawning', of 'insight', of 'seeing' a psychological connection. I have already drawn attention to the interchangeability between 'soul', 'spirit' and 'wind'. I was seeking to convey some mysteries to men whose lives were dominated by practical matters. However, all airmen are superstitious, and the medium of the air generated its own mythology. As in psychotherapy, the problem was to address the 'true' mysteries. It was a task which came close to Winnicott's desire to unravel the true and the false self.

Vision and sight have continued to fascinate me throughout my life. The ophthalmologists I have met were mostly gifted, innovative and sometimes colourful. Squadron Leader Kelly, with whom I worked on several projects, had the sort of inventive mind that always gave hope of a solution to a problem. He, like the doctor of my brief encounter in Bedfordshire, was passionate about the war. If he came across a weak or ineffective commander, or an injustice, he would write letters to those in high places. It was even rumoured that his letters were always copied to the King. He did achieve something this way, but he was more than once up before the Director General of Medical Services, who on one occasion told him that he would have been court-martialled in peace-time. His rebellious nature served him and others well in wartime, and I identified with it, although lacking his courage of action. At Warlingham Park after the war, a colleague and I got interested in the way schizophrenics saw their world. We wondered whether they saw things differently with their right and left eyes, and we conducted numerous experiments in the hospital dark room to test this. In the course of this we went to see a somewhat eccentric but fascinating peer, whose name I now forget, who took us to lunch at Brooke's Club and afterwards spent the afternoon discussing the eye and its visual problems. After tea he took us to his garage where two magnificent Edwardian cars were gleaming. It was a remarkable day out for two young psychiatrists in training, and his generosity towards us is rare today. Much later I came across the celebrated Dr Philip Inman who at the age of 90 was still visiting the eye clinic at the Queen Alexandra Hospital, Portsmouth. His life work lay in linking psychodynamics and ophthalmology. He studied the common stye, for example, known as the *hordoleum*, or grain of barley. His belief that there is a close connection between the development of a stye and the reproductive process appears naïve, but was well founded in practice. I persuaded him to come and lecture to the medical and nursing staff at Knowle Hospital, where he cited case after case in support of his ideas. The last I saw of him that day was sitting on a low stool with a circle of registrars literally at his feet. It took me back to a vision of Hippocrates and his cedar tree on the island of Kos, nearly two and a half millennia earlier.

I link those beginnings with my feelings that there are always two ways of looking at the world. Eddington (1929) wrote: 'I have settled down to the task of writing these lectures and have drawn up my chairs to two tables.' (p.xi) His two tables were his familiar table, which he described as 'substantial', and his scientific table, which he describes as 'mostly emptiness. Sparsely scattered in that emptiness are numerous electrical charges rushing about with great speed...yet it supports my writing paper as satisfactorily as table No. 1' (p.xii). I also have my two 'tables'. My No. 1 is the familiar worldly object. My No. 2 table is my dream-table, the table of my visions, like a table painted by an impressionist artist. As time has passed I have placed less reliance on the apparent certainty afforded by reality, and more on the psychic realities of dreams and visions. As a schizophrenic patient of long ago put it, 'I am driving along and see a cyclist ahead, and I never know whether to steer round him or drive straight through him. They are both the same.'

A patient who felt that her life was barren in the extreme had an extravagant dream-life. The dreams might be of rich banquets, of a theatre where the secrets of life were being enacted, of an oasis in the desert. But she was always denied acceptance into this dream world; she had to leave the banquet, or she was behind a pillar and so could not see the play. Thus she had undervalued reality and longed for her dream world to be actualised. Yet the dream world contained the material for her release, which she achieved only after several years of turbulent living, and some time after her therapy with me had ended.

My reflections on this crucial transitional phase of my life lead me to conclude that my drive had been, from my earliest days, to penetrate the mystery and at the same time to keep the mystery. The world has not proved big enough to allow us to see its unknown places as our forebears did. The myths of Prester John in the Middle Ages, and of 'darkest Africa' in more recent times, have lost their power. I fell under their spell, but my real love was the vastness of the heavens, transferred as a student into the mysteries of the human body, and again, in the RAF, into the alien world of the upper atmosphere and the darkness of the night sky. In all of these, it is the same eye which is viewing the universe at one moment, and moving to the solid reality of the telescope the next. It was a small step from here to my fascination with the mysteries of the unconscious. Arthur Eddington (1929), in the introduction to his Gifford lectures (1927), wrote that he had two tables, but he could only 'see' one; the other was a scientific and mathematical concept. My own dreams are visual and I 'see' them, but I cannot see my patient's dreams. To understand them, I had to have a framework, just as Eddington had his scientific framework. Although I decided early on that Jung offered a framework with which I could resonate, I was also seeking my own as well.

Many books have been written by those attempting to make this scientific table understandable in terms of our everyday experience. Similarly, many volumes also exist whose intention is to give meaning to the language and the imagery of the unconscious. The outpourings of both disciplines have passed beyond the students of these subjects into the national consciousness via biography, novels and the media. The results of this process undergo changes of emphasis and content according to the ebb and flow of social and cultural values. Popular books of the 1930s emphasised the power of the instincts, especially the 'sex instinct', and devoted much space to 'sublimation'. The subject of Freudian slips of the tongue and unconscious forgetting were derived from his book *The*

Psychopathology of Everyday Life (Freud 1953–1974). During the 20th century the Oedipal complex has been alternately worked to death or ridiculed, along with the whole concept of infantile sexuality. Jung's classification of psychological types achieved popularity after the Second World War at a time when clinical psychologists such as Allport were writing extensively about the subject. Jung's deeper studies of the collective unconscious have proved too great a mystery for most, but nevertheless our language has been enriched by the common use of concepts such as 'anima', 'animus', 'archetype' and 'mandala'. Adler has not had much of a look in recently. The post-Freudians have made their mark. Bowlby raised human awareness of the process of early attachment, while Winnicott raised the status of children, and showed, through books like *The Piggle* (1980) how the intuition of the therapist can be recognised by a child, and used in promoting the transference. Object relations theory has permitted us all to play with ideas derived from projection and introjection, Bateson gave us the double bind, Maslow the peak experience; the list is long.

The derivatives of the various schools of analysis have spawned a vast number of 'movements' in the fields of individual therapy, family therapy and group therapy. The cult that decrees that everybody can have everything has resulted in 'counselling' being offered for almost every conceivable emotional disturbance without a clear knowledge of whether it does good. At the other end of the scale there is a vast number of people whose neurosis requires skilled psychotherapeutic help who receive little. They frequent doctors' surgeries, they throng the out-patient clinics of our hospitals, and they are regular attendees at psychiatric clinics. At the latter they are more likely to receive drugs than psychotherapy. In all these respects the analytic movement can be likened to religion. The Church maintains the central tenets of the faith and its liturgy. It trains the priests, its practitioners and heirs to the apostolic succession. Similarly, all through the 20th century, the mainstream of Freudian and Jungian practitioners have kept the faith of their respective founders. They have developed healthily, and the old rivalry and mutual distrust has been replaced in recent years by much interchange of views. Training institutes have emerged, and each of the main disciplines has several subgroups with their own training programmes. The training is generally rigorous and accordingly psychoanalysis in its various forms remains the province of the few and its purchase expensive.

In the years after the war I struggled to adapt my chosen speciality to my image of the ideal doctor which I had carried for years. It was that of the doctor-naturalist; the explorer of the human condition; the one who depended on first principles. Those first principles were to do with the way the body is put together and how it functions. Now another and vital category of first principles was within my grasp, that of the mind. However, I decided that I could not possibly abandon six years of the study of medicine, followed by five years of intense physiological work, in favour of the single-minded study and practice of Jungian analytical psychology, seductive though this idea was. The result was the years of transitional phases and my search for a model which I have already described in Chapters 2, 3 and 4.

I discovered quite early that I viewed medicine and therapy differently from most of my colleagues. In the case of electro-convulsive therapy (ECT), for example, they were only interested in the effects of the treatment whereas I was concerned with the experience of the patient. From my notes made in 1950:

> Mrs C.W. aged 34. The breakdown which led to her hospital admission was of six weeks' duration, although she had not been entirely free from psychotic symptoms for five years. She thought that her husband was trying to electrocute her, that he was trying to turn her into an animal, degrading her and making her into a prostitute. During the war she had had an affair with a German, by whom she had had a child. When I interviewed her she had been in hospital for six weeks and had had six ECTs, the last being three weeks previously. Her husband was said to have had several psychotic breakdowns.
>
> She told me that she feared the treatment greatly, and believed that it was an exhibition of the part on the Germans, whom she supposed to have been victorious, to torture her for cowardice as an Englishwoman. Her heroes are Germanic, or Indian. She spoke of her childhood when she had aspirations to do good in the world; she wanted to travel abroad and help lame dogs and minorities, and she wanted to marry an Indian. As her frustrated desires developed in fantasy during her teens and during the war she fell in love with her German ideal, for whom she would be prepared to die. She wants many children, preferably by foreigners, and they must all be twins. She believes her lover was a twin, and that she had twins by him, but that one died.
>
> Her attitude to me was highly ambivalent. She thought I was clever, but also a potential torturer. She believed that I had administered ECT to her, which was not the case. She asked me whether I was going to kill her. She thought I was a foreigner, perhaps German or Japanese. ECT she said was turning her into an animal, and thus away from her high ideals and aspirations.

Looking at these notes today I am struck by the creative potential in her desire to have numerous twins by her hero-lovers. She was, however, living in the narrow world afforded by the suburbs of Croydon, married to a psychologically disabled husband and responsible for their children. Psychosis was the only outlet for such energy. What my colleagues were trying to do was to destroy the very forces which, if they could have been integrated into her personality, would have changed her life.

I was trying to raise the status of thought disorder and depression, not only in the perception of the patient, but also by those who were close to the patient and above all by their doctors. I addressed this question in a paper (R.A. Sandison

1972), to which I made a reference in a different context in the last chapter. I wrote:

> Depression…is a thin word, declaring a position of hopelessness and despair. It contrasts with the ancient, emotive melancholy, the 'black humour', for, as a 16th century physician put it, 'melancholy occupies the mind and changes the temperature of it'. (From Hunter and McAlpine 1963.) Melancholy or words of similar meaning occur in most literature and medical writings from earliest times. It was a constant condition of man, contrasted with joy and equated with sin, guilt, disaster and annihilation. Melancholy and sadness were the constant companions of some men, for others it was elevated to unusual heights. (p.1227)

After discussing at some length my views concerning the nature of depression and describing some current social and cultural attitudes towards it, I continued:

> Those people who suffer from disorders of their personalities and who are rarely depressed may appear to others to be unapproachable, difficult to understand and difficult to get to know … In psychotherapy the presence of depression often affords the only way through to the real person beneath a mass of defensive attitudes. To be depressed may be to undertake the dark night of the soul, or, as Jung has described it, the night journey under the sea. But, out of the chaos of hell, positive and healing forces arise. Not only does he who undertakes this journey emerge permanently transformed, but rebirth may not be possible any other way. In simple terms, those who have come through the pit of depression and the temptations of self-destruction are those who know death, but they also know life more abundantly. Those who have worked through a severe depression with the help of another person need not fear again, for their joy will be greater in future and their depression never again so severe. (p.1229)

It was a very confident statement, and one based on my own experience of treating patients with depression. Looking back, I almost certainly had my mother's depression and the manner of her recovery held as a model quite unconsciously. I also recall that my studies of the patients admitted to Warlingham Park Hospital in the 1920s had shown that almost all severe depressives recovered within a year. The therapeutic aids were good nursing in hospital, adequate diet and creative occupation. Fashions change but good psychotherapy has the same components of caring, with the added bonus of gaining self-knowledge. The last paragraph of my paper reads:

> Ten years ago doctors were convinced that the message to lay helpers such as social workers and clergy was that depressed people were ill and not sinful or bad. Psychotherapists and many social workers are now concerned that too many depressives are seen as sick and therefore treated with drugs or ECT. In extolling the virtues of ECT many doctors have lost sight of the value of psychotherapy in depression and the help which social workers and voluntary organisations can give to depressives. (p.1229)

Psychiatry has been bedevilled by the medical model, which describes all that comes the psychiatrist's way as 'illness', and therefore of biological origin, requiring medicinal treatment. The resort to drugs is interpreted by the patient as a 'brush-off', a disregard for his or her distress and inner feelings.

In the early sixties I was approached by a colleague, a pathologist, who had come to a full stop, being unable to work or take on any professional responsibility. He was 49 years of age, the age at which his father had died suddenly from a coronary attack. I knew his wife and family well, and what a secure home they had created. I arranged for him to stay at home, and for him to be cared for and cosseted in every way, with no anxieties, telephone calls or demands made on him. I visited every day and spent time with him. I forget whether he received anti-depressants, which did not seem important. Under this regime he gradually recovered, and went on to lead a useful and satisfying life. In this therapeutic approach I was more like the Victorian physicians, such as Hilton, whose book *Rest and Pain* (1987) was still in vogue when I was a student. In acting as I did the naturalist in me was at work.

Animals and the natural world figure quite prominently in my dreams. About the time we moved to Ledbury I dreamt that Beth and I were living in a house with a cat and a garden. I am in the garden, Beth is in the house with the cat, and I am talking to a pair of wrens. The male bird asks if they can make their nest in the house. I say this will be quite all right, but I will have to consult the cat first. The birds take refuge in my pocket and we go into the house where a house martin is already nesting. Beth and the cat both think that it is a good idea for the wrens to stay. Not all my dreams about animals have this cosy and romantic feel, but I introduce it to indicate that I see all life as a continuum. I like talking to animals, and they give me their wisdom from time to time. In our real garden spiders are among my favourites, about which most people, of course, are ambivalent. I meet the large cats in Shetland. In 1975 I have to find a way of combating a 'team of lions', which I do by a process of simple cunning. In 1986 I meet a lioness and a tiger in Shetland, and in another dream, a snow leopard which is friendly. In 1995, when I was reflecting on matters of consciousness, I dreamt that I meet a rather proud-looking lion in Shetland. We had a relationship, but it was important that we keep our distance.

Of course analysts could read other interpretations into these dreams. I offer them here to emphasise how the unconscious is closer knit to the rest of creation than we allow.

There has been a resurgence of feeling for a naturalist approach to medicine recently. A leader in *The Lancet* (Editorial, 1999) refers to the likelihood that public trust in doctors is waning, and asks whether there is a way back up. The writer quotes an essay by John Ryle entitled *The Physician as Scientist and Naturalist*, given to the Cambridge University Medical Society in 1931. He remarked that the experimental geniuses of Harvey and Lister laid the foundations for Western medicine, and Ryle argued that, even in his day, contemporaries 'all too often forget the mortar necessary to support these foundations' (p.1485). The doctor, he writes, is first and foremost a student of nature, observing, recording, classifying and analysing. *The Lancet* leader quotes him as saying 'the naturalistic temperament and the physicianly temperament are, as we should imagine, close relations, if not identical twins' (p.1485). The article concludes: 'A naturalistic emphasis does have one advantage – it reveals the importance of time and experience in the practice of doctoring, qualities now often forgotten or even derided'. (p.1485)

The physiologist Claude Bernard, early in the 20th century, gave medicine the concept of the *milieu interior* which emphasised that the physiological mechanisms of the body maintained it in a constant state. If the blood sugar drops, the liver immediately converts some of its stored glycogen into more glucose. If we get cold, we seek warmth or shiver to keep our body temperature constant. The pH of the blood is kept constant by buffer mechanisms. I have long been interested as much in the constancy of the physical state of our planet as I am in its disturbances. The proportion of gases in our atmosphere has remained almost constant for centuries, and even now there is some uncertainty as to whether all our carbon emissions are altering the milieu significantly. As Anthony Storr (1999) has pointed out, Jung applied this principle of self-regulation to the mind. The idea that the unconscious maintains the mental *status quo* raises all sorts of possibilities. The most reassuring of these is that the unconscious is always on our side. One of the watchwords of group analysis is 'trust the group', by which we mean that we should trust the wisdom and regulating power of the group matrix, which is the interconnected stream of unconscious elements from all its members. In therapy we may rightly challenge the ego splits and faulty assumptions of our patient, but we challenge or misinterpret the unconscious at our peril.

The interesting question arises as to whether we can make the same assumptions when working with a psychotic patient. What appear to the therapist as distortions of reality are dear to the patient. If we destroy them with drugs the patient is convinced that we are not on his side. If we challenge them in therapy we take the same risks of alienating our patient as we do when we misinterpret a dream of a non-psychotic patient. It is only the patient's own experience which he regards as familiar and 'normal'. I have already described (Chapter 3) how my psychotic patient Patrick believed that he could charge himself up from the spark plugs of his car. Patrick told us in a group that he had once met someone who claimed that he could walk on the River Thames. 'Of course I knew he was mad.' It is the clash between the patient's own psychotic system and reality which has to be addressed if he is not to live a life of alienation from other people. We are much more anxious about the patient whose psychotic thinking tells him, or commands him, to kill someone, for example. It was this kind of consideration that has led me to assert that psychotic patients mostly come to our notice for social reasons. It is as if the psychotic patient has developed his own secondary self-regulatory system, and that our task is to help him to search for the lost one.

Writing this in the closing months of the 20th century I continue to consider the way in which social change affects the development of consciousness in the West. In a paper written in 1993 (Sandison 1995) I aired this. I commenced with Jung's comment that we could not have understood the writings of the mediaeval alchemists prior to this century because there was no psychology of the unconscious (Jung 1954). However, it is unlikely that the alchemists ever really believed in the literal transmutation of base metals into gold, which seems to me to be a product of 19th century materialism. They had their own reasons for veiling the mysteries of the unconscious, and the Middle Ages, particularly the 12th century, was a time of deep introspection and romantic thought. Colin Morris (1972) examines the mediaeval search for self-knowledge and for a psychology to understand the nature of human feelings. He wrote:

> The desire for self-knowledge lay also behind the keen interest which the twelfth century showed in psychology, an interest felt by many different groups. Fashionable society's enthusiasm for the subject was reflected in the inclusion in the romances of passages devoted to the discussion of psychology. In the Cligés of Chrétien de Troyes, the two lovers of the first half of the novel, Alexander and Soredamors, indulge in lengthy self-questioning about the nature of their feelings for each other, and there are some austere sections about the meaning of common terms – what is meant by giving one's 'heart' to another? There was, therefore, a wide concern about psychology, which was also evident in the number of scholars who attempted a thorough examination of the subject. The starting point here, as so often, was the work of Augustine. (p.76)

I wrote this paper on consciousness in the 20th century in the months after Louis Zinkin, my analyst during 1984–1988, had died. Like Foulkes, he had died while conducting a group. It was a couples group led jointly with his wife Hindle. I owe so much to him. During analysis there were points of contact to which he would refer with shy relish from time to time. He enjoyed my cricketing metaphor about the greatest reward in the game coming from hitting a ball over the boundary. He liked my telling him that if you wanted good fishing at sea you would sometimes have to go where the water was roughest. Then there were the two paths which led to the same place but by different routes. And, of course, the time when I asked my mother when she was going to get better. He would refer to these with a shy smile, as if we were two schoolboys sharing a secret. This disarming manner assured me of the mutual respect we had for the secrets we shared. It is indeed with some anxiety that I share them here. One always hopes that the gods will not be offended. There was an acknowledgement of the fact that we were both exiles, although from very different settings. I wrote an obituary for Louis for the Bulletin of the Group Analytic Society. It was one of many tributes to him. And the following year there was a memorial evening at the Royal College of Music which celebrated his life and his love of music. I cannot say more that others have not said, except to say that I loved him and I treasure his writings. The latter were collected and edited by Hindle Zinkin and others (Zinkin, Gordon and Haynes 1998).

The desire of the Greek physicians that man should know himself is reflected in the teaching of the desert fathers of the 2nd and 3rd centuries. They taught that a man who desired to talk to God through prayer and other means had first to know himself – that is, to know who that person was who was making the prayer. Sadly, in many of our churches today, most of the prayers are not about ourselves, who remain unknown, but dwell on the miserable state of mankind, mostly in countries remote from our own. We therefore need to examine whether the psychological insights of the 20th century are real, or variants on ancient themes driven by social change.

In my paper referred to above I suggested that there had been a 'massive growth of consciousness during this century' (Sandison 1995, p.340). On reflection I am not so sure. What I believe has happened is that there has been a shift from outer to inner. Our Victorian forebears were exploring the world. Freud and Jung in this century turned our thinking to our inner nature. By 1900 man's image of the world had already expanded to an astonishing degree. Humanity was not a separate creation, we were part of the whole living kingdom. The world was millions of years old, and not created in 4004 BC. At the same time the Earth was shrinking. 'Darkest Africa' had been explored, the conquest of the polar regions was near, and the British Empire stretched across the globe.

The 20th century brought new means of communication and travel. I grew up with them; they were among the exciting pleasures of my adolescence. There was a tremendous romance about the desire to go further and faster than ever before. Lindbergh and Amy Johnson's transatlantic flights, Alcock and Brown to Australia, the great motor speed trials on Daytona Beach, and, not least, the Schneider trophy air races round the Isle of Wight are all etched deeply in my memory. During the latter I was glued to the radio, savouring every sound. Likewise my imagination was stirred by hearing the first radio broadcasts from America. The voice, rising and fading through a mass of static, symbolised the very radio waves themselves and I was stirred at the romance of being a witness to the results of the limits of technology. My thirst to understand first principles, to know how things were put together and how they worked was well satisfied by that relatively new and still wonderful machine, the motor car. With a few tools and the help of the local garage owner and my father's friends I soon learned how to strip down a motor engine, as one could in those days.

In these ways my personal mental growth kept pace with the pace of events. The latter were still in tune with age-old deposits in the human psyche. I felt refreshed and calmed by them. What *was* new and disturbing was the new physics and the new psychology. These, together with the associated changes in social thinking, practice and mores, have added another layer to human consciousness, which has displaced much that Western man brought with him into the 20th century. This has led to an imbalance between the ancient wisdom of the unconscious and modern consciousness.

Freud was fond of turning things on their head. Of God, he said, in effect: 'For millennia man has thought of himself as being made in the image of God, but what if, instead, God was made in the image of man'(author's interpretation). It is an intriguing exercise, but the problem is that it leads to nihilism, which has characterised so much of 20th century thought. We tamper with age-old myths at our peril. The scientists played similar games with the consequences of the theory of relativity. James Jeans' proposition that a kettle of water *might* boil when placed on a block of ice is a nice theoretical idea, but of no practical significance. Ideas like this have nevertheless become woven into our late 20th century thinking and politics. The huge consequences of the BSE scare, claiming as it has a tiny proportion of victims, is perhaps a social derivative of Jeans' kettle.

Freud published *The Interpretation of Dreams* in 1900 (Freud 1953–1974). Jung took his time, and claimed that he would not publish on dreams until he had studied 20,000 of them, which he did in 1916 (Jung 1916). The cataclysm of the First World War was then at its height. During and after the war psychoanalysis became a tool for assisting those who were the victims of battle neurosis, then known as 'shell-shock'. It was a condition that could affect any soldier, of whatever social class or rank. Yet another Victorian myth, that it was mostly those of 'poor stock' who succumbed to mental breakdown, was being demolished.

The work of W.H. Rivers at Ravenscraig Military Hospital for Officers during the war, and that of Crichton Miller who founded the Tavistock Clinic after the war, brought the realities of psychotherapy as a valid treatment into national consciousness. It was the beginning of a movement which has spread right through the remainder of the century – a desire to find wholeness and to seek alternatives to conventional religion and moral values. The religious movements of the 1930s were mostly evangelical, emphasising 'conversion' on the Pauline model to Christianity. Once 'saved', you did not need to do much more. In Kipling's story *On the Gate, '16,* (1926), St Peter at the gates of heaven, far from questioning each new arrival, is sending out envoys to round up the hordes of men, victims of the Battle of the Somme, before the devil could get his hands on them. And in the 1960s the world discovered that LSD and other hallucinogenic drugs appeared to open the gates to a 20th century paradise.

There have always been those who were enlightened by the wisdom and preoccupations of their own generation, and there have always been the half-alive majority, for whom their relatively unconscious state was all they could manage. Nearly 40 years ago I had a Swedish psychiatrist as a guest who was interested to learn about our work with LSD. At its conclusion we went to Stonehenge and we sat together on one of the megaliths for a long time without speaking. He then looked round and said, 'Man has not changed much in 3000 years.' I add to that two thoughts of my own. Language is the greatest and most universally understood tool we have for communication and transmission of ideas and culture. It is the primary tool of therapy. It is language which is continually developing and changing. My colleague may have been right, man has not changed much, but his means of communication and the technology for doing so have grown immeasurably. My second thought is that psychoanalysis and its derivatives, used as a method of treatment for the troubled and disordered mind, is the only one to survive the century. Freud's *Interpretation of Dreams*, published in 1900, still has validity in the year 2000.

CHAPTER 9

A Century of Psychotherapy

Many patients who come to a psychotherapist feel that they should present a coherent biography of their lives, with special emphasis on the events of childhood. They commonly think in terms of events, but another way of presenting one's history might be to offer a list of the books and stories which made a deep impression. In my early life books were given, chosen for me; in later childhood I chose my own. In adolescence I matched those turbulent years with wide and voracious reading and some of these books were viewed with disapproval by my father. He would dismiss writers such as Shaw and Bertrand Russell with devastating one-liners, which increased my curiosity. I might reach a different conclusion. The magic of those milli-seconds of insight into his true nature and beliefs with which he had presented books during my childhood was thus obscured for many years. By good fortune we regained that sense of wonder after he retired, when we were able to recommend books to each other, and criticise our choices. We entered that world of inner experience once more with the works of Charles Williams and C.S. Lewis, Tolkien and others. It was a link with myself at the age of 10 when I had devoured the tales collected by the Brothers Grimm. *The Robber Bridegroom* (1975) particularly appealed to me and I decided to read it to my grandmother. It is a classical tale of good and evil. The miller's beautiful daughter becomes betrothed to the leader of a murderous gang of robbers, but she succeeds in witnessing their sadistic deeds. These she relates at her wedding feast as if she had dreamt them, and, in a dramatic gesture, produces a finger which the robbers had chopped off a young girl and which had fallen at her feet while she lay hidden in their cave. With this proof the robber chief was arrested, and the story ends: 'Then he and his whole troop were executed for their infamous deeds.' I never got as far as this in my reading aloud. When I got to the line which referred to the robbers' treatment of one of their victims, 'They gave her wine to drink, three glasses full, one glass of white wine, one glass of red, and a glass of yellow, and with this her heart burst in twain', grandmother stopped me and said she could not listen to such a horrible story. It was one of my great rites of passage, and I remember vividly the very room and the chair she was sitting in. I had eaten the fruit, my Garden of Eden had vanished, I had lost my innocence and was cast into a world where good and evil were no longer one, but hard and separate. There is a paradox here. As von Franz (1970) says: 'Fairy tales are the purest and simplest expression of collective unconscious psychic processes' (p.1). They were originally stories for both children and adults. By resonating with the story I was truer to the archetype than my grandmother, as children are more at home with the contents of the collective unconscious than grown-ups. This fact escaped the notice of many Victorians who carefully trimmed nastiness from their fairy tales. My grandmother, born in 1861, was a good example.

I have struggled with the idea of reconciling good and evil for much of my life. I tried to bring some of my ideas together in 1993 (Sandison 1993). This paper grew out of the group analytic workshop in 1992 which I described in Chapter 6. In the creation myth in the Book of Genesis, God initiated the separation of primal chaos into opposites: heaven and earth, light and dark, male and female. We are told that God saw this as good, and the goodness of it seems to be God's view of his creative act and its results. God took no responsibility for Adam's subsequent action in stealing the knowledge of good and evil from the Tree of Knowledge. It was man, rather than woman, who made darkness evil. However, in the parallel myth of Lilith we find that whereas Eve was created either out of pure dust or from Adam's rib, Lilith, also the first woman, was created out of 'filth and excrement' (Colonna 1980). Neither Adam, Eve or Lilith could escape this malignant contamination with evil.

Our ancestors attempted to solve the riddle of good and evil by the idea that both co-existed in man and in God. As this seemed unfair to man and discourteous to God, good and evil had to separate. Woman, of course, has paid the price ever since, being cast in the role of the temptress, the seducer, the 'power behind the throne'. Christ was only too well aware of this judgement on woman. In one of the most beautiful and moving stories in the whole Bible Christ went to dine with a Pharisee named Simon. According to St Luke, a woman, 'who had a bad name in the town', heard that Jesus was dining with the Pharisee, so she came and brought with her an alabaster jar of ointment. 'She waited behind him at his feet, weeping, and her tears fell on his feet, and she wiped them away with her hair; then she covered his feet with kisses and anointed them with the ointment.'

Not surprisingly, the Pharisee was scandalised, whereupon Christ said to him:

> Simon, you see this woman? I came into your house, and you poured no water over my feet, but she has poured out her tears over my feet and wiped them away with her hair. You gave me no kiss, but she has been covering my feet with kisses ever since I came in. You did not anoint my head with oil, but she has anointed

my feet with ointment. For this reason I tell you that her sins, her many sins, must have been forgiven her, or she would not have shown such great love. It is the man who has been forgiven little who shows little love. Then he said to her 'Your sins are forgiven'. (Luke 7: 36–38)

This was not the only situation in which Christ sought to put an end to the split between man, who took on the good, as the lawmaker and keeper of the commandments, and woman, who carried all the evil and sorrow in the world. His love and friendship for Mary Magdalene, and his condemnation of the accusers of the woman 'taken in adultery', set the scene for a religion of tolerance and forgiveness, which, sadly, has been far from being realised during most of the subsequent history of the Christian Church.

Looked at psychodynamically, the sins of the woman at Simon's house resided in her tears, which were not only incorporated into the body of Christ, but were also wiped away by her act of repentance. Freed from her burden she could express her love with her kisses and her union with Christ in the anointing. Psychologically, it is the process which we aim for with our patients, but for which a price has to be paid. To acknowledge our own evil, and to integrate it into our consciousness, is to end splitting, but it is a painful and lengthy process. In 1993 I wrote:

> More than forty years of working with people have slowly and painfully taught me that we can only work with the dark side of our patients if we recognise and understand the evil side of our own natures, just as we can only work effectively with psychotics if we know the madness in ourselves. The years have also taught me something else, that all patients have spiritual and religious problems, conscious or unconscious, and that we, as therapists…need a religious stance ourselves if we are to meet these spiritual needs, which, taken in the mass, amount to a vast hunger. (p.212)

My desire to do what I could to meet some of this 'vast hunger' led me to seek personal analysis in 1948. It was my first experience of being a patient rather than a doctor. The early transference images were to do with doubt about whether my analyst and I were teacher and student or fellow travellers engaged on a joint journey. I decided that I did not wish to pursue a Jungian analytical training but to find my own way alongside the mainstream of psychiatry. First I had to discover more about who I was. I had a dream that I was returning to my family house, but that my parents had moved to another house. Inside my parent's home I discovered one of my patients, and we had a session in an upper room. It was during this session that I knew that I was accompanied by a 'dark image of myself'. I was then overcome with a 'great anger' which I directed towards my patient, 'accusing her of obtuseness and of causing her husband's insanity'. It became clear to me from that time, when I discovered, so to speak, my shadow, that I had a lot of work to do on myself before I could be a good therapist.

Over 50 years later I am still learning. I still dream of two houses, but they are both now mine. The house of my parents was the house where I learned from my father's wisdom and his books; where I observed the weather and the heavens and recorded all I saw. It was where I had my laboratory, with its bench for test tubes, retorts, flasks, Bunsen burners and pipettes, the shelves for neatly labelled glass-stoppered bottles of chemicals and my notebooks, some of which survive to this day. This is the dream house where I see my first patients for therapy and discover my shadow. In my two present-day houses I live and work in one, while the other is comfortingly there as the place of research and discovery. It used to have two empty rooms on the top floor, but I have filled one of them in recent years. It has become my new laboratory where I experiment with and make books. My other room? There must always be a place for future development. The shadow – does anyone ever completely come to terms with it?

Staying close to the mainstream of psychiatry has meant that I have been a close observer of the relationship between it and the psychoanalytic schools of the 20th century. In 1947 I attended the 30th Course for the Diploma of Psychological Medicine at the Maudsley Hospital, and there was almost no mention of psychotherapy apart from a lecture by S.F. Foulkes on group analysis, neither was one likely to need any knowledge of the subject to pass the exam. Fifteen years later I met Dennis Hill at the Maudsley who spoke of the 'two psychiatries' and his desire to bring psychotherapy into the domain of mainstream psychiatry, with which I strongly resonated. In the pages of this book I have described how for years I shifted uneasily between the two, and tried without success to arrange a marriage based on LSD therapy. Despite changes in the training curriculum for the Royal College Membership exam, psychotherapy is still the poor relation of psychiatry.

A paradox is exposed when we consider patients' expectations. There is very little literature about the experiences of patients at their first psychiatric interview. Ruth Michaels (1975) saw 30 new patients for half an hour before their first psychiatric interview and again a week later with the object of discovering their expectations and whether they were realised. Some of the patients had not realised that they were going to see a psychiatrist, four thought they would be asked to lie on a couch, 13 did not find talking to the psychiatrist helpful. Some were offered tablets at the end of the interview, and one man, ECT, which he had greatly feared. A frequent complaint was that the psychiatrist seemed in a hurry or was not interested in them, and one said that in his case he was 'like a man stuck in a traffic jam in a hurry to get home to his tea'. Four psychiatrists were involved in the study.

Consequent upon Miss Michaels' report I introduced a system whereby all new patients were offered a pre-psychiatric interview with a psychiatric nurse within a week of their referral. This proved very popular and reduced the number of those who failed to attend their first interview. The fantasies and expectations of people concerning psychiatrists and their work is based on the media, films and to a lesser extent on novels. These undoubtedly produce distortions, but they are based on the reality that the couch is used by psychoanalysts, that they do enquire about fantasies and dreams, and they do offer interpretations. In reality what patients are hoping for is that the psychiatrist will be interested in them, that they will have his whole attention, uninterrupted and in a relaxed atmosphere. They also desire that the interview shall start on time, that there will be enough time, and that they will feel better at the end. The best way to achieve this is for the psychiatrist to insist that his patients have this time, and for him to adopt a strict discipline of time keeping. It happens in private practice, it is also good clinic practice.

Dr Irvine Kreeger, consultant psychotherapist at King's, addressed the Wessex Psychotherapy Society in 1975. He spent most of his talk describing the psychodynamics of an occasion when he unavoidably arrived 20 minutes late to see the first patient of an afternoon's session. It made a deep impression on all who heard him, and made me realise the importance of time which I have just emphasised. A move away from the medical model would move the two psychiatries, general and psychotherapeutic, much closer together. At the time when I was seeing 'all-comers' as distinct from patients referred for psychotherapy, I always acted on the assumption that I would be seeing them more than once. I have not taken a formal psychiatric history for many years; patients will tell you about themselves in their own way and events and people will emerge as appropriate. Nothing should be extracted from the patient; it must come out in its own time. The psychotic patient carefully guards his psychotic thoughts, fantasies and hallucinations and to extract them by direct questioning is an affront to him. Sometimes a patient new to me has arrived with a thick folder of past notes. I never read them. The patient has some reason for coming now, and it won't be found in the notes. All these matters seem straightforward and simple, but I have seen so many patients who after years of attendance at psychiatric clinics have never really felt heard, neither have their inner problems been addressed, that I feel justified in offering these few ground rules.

In 1984 I entered analysis with Louis Zinkin. I have referred to this in Chapter 6. I had recently left Shetland for London, and felt emotionally exhausted and dead. I envied Louis for his settled life in London, for having lived in the same place for a long time, and for having single-mindedly pursued Jungian analytical psychology all his professional life. He found advantages in my life, and I felt after a time that he was envious of my varied experience. It has been characteristic of my family, for many generations, to move every now and then. Two centuries or more ago it was within a radius of a few miles, today, like so much else in modern life, I increase that by a factor of a hundred. The first move was when I was four years old, from Shetland to the southern outskirts of London. We had moved from the home of father's parents to the town where my mother had been brought up and where her family lived. As recorded earlier in this book I have had many dreams about travel by sea, but those referring to Shetland are almost always about leaving there. In 1948 I dreamt that I was leaving Shetland and had a steamer ticket but no cabin. Before I can secure one a crowd of southern bureaucrats claim all of them, but the captain of the vessel is a friend of the family so I pass the night away in his domain. This dream has not altered much. In 1983 the ferry leaves without me because I am chatting to friends. In 1986 the ship is half flooded and has to be pumped out before we can sail. A coffin comes aboard, there is to be a sea-burial, perhaps it is my father's coffin. My family had lived in what are known in the South as 'those remote islands' for at least five centuries, and we have accurate records for most of the last three. However, if you had been there it was the rest of the world that was remote, such is the relativity of perception. Islands develop their own archetypes, and I cannot escape their deep imprint. It does not surprise me that, in my dreams, I find it so difficult to leave.

We moved again when I was nine years old to the outskirts of Wimbledon. This was the place where, as mentioned above, I had my telescope, my weather station and my laboratory. We left there in 1940, when the house was requisitioned, and for various reasons, the family never returned. I set up my base with my own family after the war at Warlingham, and moved to Worcester as consultant in 1951. Here there was plenty of professional scope, and I might have stayed there, in pleasant rural surroundings, for the rest of my professional life. Among the many reasons for moving from there in 1964 was my observation that many of my colleagues in all branches of medicine were showing signs of 'burn-out'. However that may be, when I look at my subsequent history, I believe that my destiny has been to initiate processes and then to let others take on the less exciting role of keeping them going through the years. The LSD programme continued for a few years after I left and then, like the fall of Rome, fell victim to external pressures. The Worcester Samaritans has survived to this day, and the Worcester Pastoral Theology Group lasted for some years. However, that is a matter of history; what mattered to me was what I was doing at the time. It flatters one's ego to know that one's innovations have taken root, but this knowledge does nothing to assuage the inner need to create something more.

I was in Southampton for 11 years, or the duration of a sunspot cycle, and then the forces which were urging me to return to Shetland became subtler and more profound than any I had experienced before or since. Whether this was a devotion to my father-ancestors or the seduction of the mother isles, or both, is debatable, but I went there in 1975. Driven in a similar direction by similar urges, I left seven years later, leaving behind the Alcohol Resource Centre, and I had paved the way for the appointment of a much-needed full-time psychiatrist. I found it rich soil for the practice of psychotherapy. This was much valued by most of the patients, grudgingly appreciated by the GPs, and opposed by the Health Board. In 1982 it was time to leave; my destiny took me to London and ten years of work in psychotherapy, reproductive medicine and work with London Diocese. All this I have enlarged on in earlier chapters, but a summary appears appropriate here.

One important result of these five phases in my professional life has been that I have become well acquainted with beginnings and endings in psychotherapy. At the beginning of my first analysis I had a dream in which I was in a cathedral facing the altar. On either side were the symbols Alpha and Omega, the beginning and the end, the first and the last. Between them, the altar represented sacrifice and redemption. Beginnings signify a creative process, and its revelations are not necessarily all sweetness and light. Sylvia Close reported (1980) that the mothers describing their new-born children used expressions such as 'horrid', 'ugly little thing', 'ugly and elderly looking', 'beautifully ugly' and 'little stranger'. The myth of beautiful motherhood and its reality are clearly very different. Similarly, the patient enters psychotherapy with very different expectations to what he or she subsequently discovers.

Some years ago a lady of 38 was referred to me for psychotherapy. After learning that she had renal polycystic disease (from which her mother had died), she decided to 'live it up', which only added to her confusion and areas of conflict. She had an affair. She became pregnant by her husband and enjoyed the birth of her first child, saying it was the greatest experience of her life. The birth of a second child was a bad experience; the magic wouldn't return. She then rejected the first child, as a symbol of her resentment against fate. After a few weeks in therapy she started to recall dreams, and was surprised on realising that she had another and different form of mental life. It was about this time, three or four weeks into therapy, that she became rather euphorically engaged in the process.

Some weeks later she had a dream that she was climbing up a slippery cliff, against a waterfall. She was determined to make it to the top, which she did. Her comment: 'It is the turning point in my life.' Bearing in mind that the euphoria over the birth experience with her first child, 12 years earlier, had also been a 'turning point', I was wary. She then had a dream about an adder, which terrified her. She remembered that as a child she often had dreams that she was in trouble, and that her friends came to help her in the form of serpents. She then launched into a discussion about sex, and how she was determined that she would do everything she could to preserve her daughter's virginity. In the next session she reported a dream in which Chinese communists were pursuing her and her husband. They climbed a rocky mountain to get away, their guide being a blind child who knew the way perfectly. She started to improve from that time. Following the blind instincts of her child proved more healing than the euphoria of isolated achievements.

This therapy lasted only about seven months, and her case is selected fairly randomly from among several hundred. It illustrates only one of many ways in which patients become engaged in the therapeutic process and with the therapist. From the point of view of the unconscious there is little difference between seven months and seven years in therapy, but it matters greatly to the patient. He or she nearly always wants to know, 'How long?' The fact that I cannot answer this question troubles the patient, coming as it does from the doctor who is supposed to know the answer to everything. If, as probably happened with the patient quoted above, the healing forces can be shifted from their own and the therapist's omnipotence to the wisdom of the unconscious, in this case, the wisdom of a blind child, a huge shift will have taken place. It marks the creation of a therapeutic alliance in which both agree that this is the way. For this process to occur at all the patient and therapist must suit each other.

I have taken on a number of patients who have been in analysis previously. It raises the question of whether analysis ever ends. I have heard it described as a 'life sentence'. This suggests an idea of containment within a straightjacket of an analytical process which never ends, whereas at best the patient continues to explore and make use of the infinite resources of the unconscious for the rest of his life. Nevertheless, even when this happens, and perhaps because of it, he or she may feel the need for further therapy. Sometimes the patient moves or the analyst moves or dies. It is clearer cut for the therapist. Sooner or later he and his patient have to end the intimate process of their journey together. In my analysis with Louis, I had dreams of approaching a railway terminus which signalled to both of us that it was time to end. In the last dream of that sequence I meet a Jew as I am approaching Victoria Station, who takes me by the hand and we make good progress. A woman wrenches my hand free and herself takes my hand. We have an exchange about which of us is a detective. In my next dream I leave Shetland for the last time, I shall never go there again, it is painful and I am crying. But this dream of leaving Shetland, again for the last time, is repeated three nights later, when I am taking leave of my oldest and closest friend there. Finally, I am going to hospital in an ambulance with my first wife, Evelyn, who is dying after the accident which in fact led to her death. Then I dream that Louis and I are going to a gathering after our last analytic session, where there will be good friendship and conversation. I find that I cannot get close to him as there are other people around. Ending therapy is a painful event, and does not always give the hoped-for sense of liberation, as I think I have shown.

I had a good ending with Louis, but sometimes, especially when one moves, it proves impossible to resolve transference problems. At best, the transference and the analytical relationship is never completely dissolved, and sometimes the bonds it creates take many years to resolve. It does, however, sometimes exhibit acute symptoms expressed in a powerful desire to follow the analyst, anger at his apparent abandonment of his patient, or the acting out of fantasies about him. There is no solution to this, and time and circumstance usually help to diminish this painful state of affairs. Some years ago, at the end of the summer break, one of my patients expressed his extreme anger with me for abandoning him for so long. His fantasy was that he wanted to take me to a monastic cell where we would remain together for ever (he was an ex-monk). It was as well that this occurred in the middle of analysis and not at its end. A number of my former patients write to me at Christmas, some of them at some length, so that I have had the privilege of knowing how they fared for many years after ending therapy. Sometimes, after a gap of a good many years, patients have returned for a visit. In those cases we have always met with pleasure, curiosity and interest, but we have always been aware that we have both changed. I do not recall a single instance in which either of us felt that it was appropriate to resume therapy, even though my patient might be aware of his need for more.

One of the themes of this book has been that the dynamic ideas derived from Freud and Jung have had a powerful and enduring influence on almost every branch of Western human endeavour throughout the 20th century. This is not the place to examine or speculate any further about the influence of psychoanalysis on the arts and sciences, liberal and academic. Many others have done this already. I propose to confine myself to the therapeutic value and use of psychotherapy.

I have tried to include the whole range of psychiatric conditions in this book. They are all amenable to psychotherapy in one form or another, provided that the setting is appropriate. Sadly, despite the fact that psychoanalysis as a form of treatment has lasted throughout the century, while other treatments have come and gone, only a small proportion of psychiatric patients receive psychotherapeutic aid. This is despite the fact that, according to Holmes (1996) in 'Psychoanalysis: An endangered species',

> Psychotherapies have proliferated, there are more than 400 at the latest count. Psychotherapy is established as mainstream treatment for many psychiatric disorders; family intervention in schizophrenia, cognitive behavioural therapy and interpersonal therapy for depression, behavioural treatments for phobic disorders among others. Research in psychotherapy has blossomed and many psychotherapeutic treatments can convincingly claim to be part of 'evidence based medicine'. (p.321)

How, therefore, does it come about that the author sees psychotherapy as an 'endangered species', and that so few patients receive its benefits? Jeremy Holmes, who wrote with some euphoria in 1996, is much less confident in his recent papers. He is a consultant psychotherapist in the NHS, and has become aware of all the traps created by the seductions of the worship of 'evidence based medicine', and the gods of cost-effectiveness and numbers of patients treated. In 1998 he wrote: 'If psychiatry is the Cinderella of medicine, psychotherapy in the

National Health Service is often the Cinderella of Cinderellas' (p.65). He goes on to state that the recently published NHS Executive document *The Future of Psychotherapy Services* (Parry and Richardson 1996) is a determined and impressive attempt to document and to address this. A reading of the document did not reassure me to the same extent. The authors had difficulty in defining what is meant by the term 'psychotherapy' in the current usage of its numerous providers. They classified it in three groups:

Type A: Psychological treatment taking place at the same time as 'other', presumably pharmacological, treatments. It is defined rather obscurely as: 'A psychological treatment as an integral component of mental health care.'

Type B: Eclectic psychological therapy and counselling.

Type C: Formal psychotherapies. Examples given are psychoanalysis, cognitive-behavioural and systemic.

Psychotherapy, in the sense that I understand it, is therefore only to be found in a small corner of these definitions. Therapeutic communities get only a single mention in the whole report, and that is by name, without any context. There is no mention of group psychotherapy as a separate mode of psychotherapy either in the section on history or elsewhere. Despite these shortcomings, the fact that it was commissioned at all is encouraging, and there is no doubt that psychotherapy exists to an extent today in the health service which was unthinkable 30 years ago. Holmes (1998) sums up the report:

The main recommendations of the report are that psychotherapy services should be comprehensive, co-ordinated, user-friendly, safe, clinically effective and cost effective. In an attempt to focus on the two latter requirements, a parallel volume *What Works for Whom?* (Roth and Fogany 1996), also commissioned by the NHSE, provides a comprehensive which-type guide to the evidence for the effectiveness of different types of psychotherapy in the main psychiatric disorders. (p.65)

An indicator of the state of psychotherapy in the NHS is the fact that there are a large number of vacancies for consultant general psychiatrists, and none for senior registrars in psychotherapy nor for consultant psychotherapists. This would suggest that the profession would become much more attractive if dynamic psychotherapy was truly an integral and central component in the training of psychiatrists. It is what doctors themselves wish and it is certainly what the public would wish to experience.

Rees (1999) reviewed his own experience as a registrar when he was invited to co-lead a therapy group with a consultant psychotherapist. He describes this as a valuable and enriching part of his training experience. He adds: 'Current deficits in training relate more to the supply of opportunities and supervision rather than low demand from trainees' (p.102). Rees quotes previous surveys which showed that the percentage of trainees receiving training and supervision in group analysis varied from 9 per cent (Arnott *et al.* 1993) to 58 per cent (Hwang and Drummond 1996). In the 1970s, when I was consultant psychotherapist in Southampton, each of the registrars spent six months with the day hospital and department of psychotherapy. In this setting they received supervised training in a therapeutic community setting, including group analytic and individual therapy. Several undertook the one year Introductory Course in Group Analysis run by the Institute of Group Analysis (London). This involved a weekly journey to London. I ran a weekly optional group for all the registrars in training in the region, which again involved some of them coming some distance, but the group usually had from ten to twelve members.

I mention this in order to draw some conclusions about training in psychotherapy. It can only be carried out adequately in areas where there is a hospital-based consultant psychotherapist. Exceptions are in those regions where university-based training programmes are in place, as at Sheffield. Here, in the words of the Director of Psychotherapy Services, Raymond Haddock (1999), 'The Specialist Psychotherapy Directorate of Community Health, Sheffield, provides a range of specialist services, including psycho-analytical and group-analytical psychotherapy, cognitive-behavioural therapy, relationship and sexual dysfunction and eating disorders to Sheffield and increasingly to surrounding districts'. (p.39)

Training in psychotherapy thus makes greater demands on both trainee and supervisor. It involves much greater participation with patients and its interactive properties with both patients and supervisors is both stimulating and demanding. It is also likely that training will, in most areas, involve some travel. The shortage of good supervisors is a serious bar to effective training, and needs to be addressed. It is clear that progress is being made, but the pages of the mainstream psychiatric journals are woefully short of articles with any hint of a psychodynamic flavour.

Throughout this book are to be found memories. I look back on my earliest years at several different levels, and one which becomes more and more prominent in my memory is 'stories, and stories and stories'. Shetland, where my ancestors lived for at least five centuries, is a meeting place of cultures, Norseman and Celt came there to live, to trade, to claim and dispute land, and to raise families. Over the centuries trade by sea came from all the states bordering the North Sea. From the late 15th century the Scots, noted for their oppression and greed, infiltrated the islands and appropriated most of the land. All brought their language, folklore and legends with them. As I have shown in my biography of my ancestor Christopher (Sandison 1997) learning and education were prime concerns. Christopher had an intense curiosity about natural phenomena, people and the whole cycle of birth, growth, maturity and death with which I strongly identify. There were always stories; stories which were handed down and with which I grew up. Thus I was introduced at an early age to the fact of good and evil. In this mythological world, good did not always triumph. I remember a roofless house being pointed out when I was quite young, as being one where the man who built it had played cards with the devil and lost, the penalty being that there would never be a roof on that house. Such tales were legion. Others concerned tales of two brothers, the archetypal version having been collected by the Grimm brothers. This complex tale of envy, jealousy, good and evil ends with the words of the younger brother: 'Then he knew how true his brother had been.' This story, in various forms, exists all over the world. In Shetland there is an island called Egilsay which was inherited by two brothers who could not agree how to divide it. Whereupon the devil raised a great storm which divided it unequally so that the brother who disputed the matter most received the least. Here the devil was on the side of justice, a role not unknown to him. One of my earlier ancestors, a centenarian born in 1681, is said to have come upon two brothers disputing how to divide a baulk of timber they had found on the shore. Christopher, who was said to have possessed great strength, split it in two with his bare hands, and solved the problem. That story has passed down the generations ever since, and has endowed Christopher with heroic qualities, and given rise to the legend of the strength of the 'Sandison wrist'. All these stories invoke magic for their fulfilment, and they always evoked magic in the telling.

I heard these stories from my family. I had no brothers or sisters, and my cousins became my siblings. The closest was Kenneth, and we were so alike that we were usually taken for brothers when together. To me he was a twin, although he was three years older than I. In my childhood fantasies we could easily have been abandoned at birth, and brought up, like Romulus and Remus, by a she-wolf. Their legend concerning the founding of Rome always fascinated me, and it puzzled me that only one twin could succeed, the other had to die. I reflected much later that Kenneth had rather a sad and unfulfilled life, and died prematurely, true to the archetype after all. My world was alive with stories of children without parents, Mowgli, the Railway Children, the Five Children and It, and others. Kenneth and I inhabited that world. We invented a secret language with which to communicate with each other exclusively.

I have already brought Kenneth into this history through his three prophetic dreams. In our late teens we spent every summer travelling together. In 1937 we decided to make an extended tour of Europe. We spent several days at Misurina, in the foothills of the Italian Alps. A young girl of about 12 spent almost all day wandering round the hills above this small town, singing the most beautiful and evocative folk songs. They filled me with sadness and longing, for she was telling the story of her people. I did not have to hear the actual words to know this. This experience in Italy has stayed with me, and after the war I realised that when listening to a patient, there is another story to be heard at a deeper level than the one of which he or she is conscious. It is my intuitive rapport with that story that enables me to make the links which release insight in my patient.

My story has a sequel. Forty years later Kenneth lay dying of cancer of the lung. Although scarcely able to speak, we started talking about those times, long ago, before the war changed everything, when we travelled and camped together. Suddenly he said: 'Do you remember...the girl that sang?' It was a moment of rapport which brought our whole lives together into the capsule of that instant. As happens with one's patients, the sharing of an experience of long ago, never mentioned before, released us both from the bondage of secrets. Indeed, he died a few days later. Before I left on that day he asked me to go into the garage and disconnect the battery on his car. What a metaphor for disengagement! As I write this I reflect on the wish that more of our therapeutic relationships might end with such elegant metaphors.

There were other stories told me by an aunt, about the origins of the world, and dinosaurs, and the planets and time, and about Newton and gravity, Harvey and the circulation of the blood, the evolution of plants and animals, and much, much more. My grandmother was carried away by Carter and the discovery of the tomb of Tutankhamun in 1922. A few years later, when we went to the British museum together, the only section I wanted to see was the Egyptian one. There my memory centres around the sun-dried mummy of an ancient Egyptian, lying naked in the sand as he might have done in death 3000 years ago. The monuments and the hieroglyphs and the Rosetta Stone were marvels, but none touched me in the way that this fragile image of humanity allowed me to glimpse something close to the origins of all stories and of human life itself.

In *Memories, Dreams, Reflections*, Jung (1961) asserted that, in writing about his earliest years, he could only 'tell stories'. 'Whether they are true or not is not my problem. The only question is whether what I tell is *my* fable, *my* truth' (p.17). I do not see my early life quite in the same way. We rewrite our own histories, but the stories and events of my early life really happened. My difficulty is to know which aspect of them is relevant to my subsequent life's work. Some would say, all of them; I offer them as part of the context for the material in this book.

The context which gives the human psyche meaning is time. We cannot be sure yet whether the 20th century is part of the industrial era, or we are sinking towards a new dark age, or whether, as Jung predicted, we have entered the age of Aquarius. It is hard to find unifying ideas and philosophies. Socially the Edwardian period is a world away from that of the 1990s. Cynically, one could say that two world wars have so impoverished the West that we have only been able to build a short-term tinselly sort of structure to replace the losses. There may be other contenders, but I rate psychoanalysis and its derivatives as being one of the most, if not *the* most, unifying influences on the human spirit in those hundred years. It has grown and diversified, it has challenged orthodox religion, but it has given meaning to much of human behaviour that was hitherto regarded as perverse or 'abnormal'. Dr Leslie MacKenzie wrote at the turn of the century (in Freud, trans. Eder, undated) that Freud had demonstrated how 'the morbid symptoms we (had previously) classified as mental diseases, had their roots in the mental processes of the normal mind' (p.vii). It was a profound change in human thinking which united 'normality' with insanity and deviance. It has had a profound effect on social policy and on our attitude towards the afflicted, and thus it characterises our century.

The scattering of the psychoanalytic community in Vienna and elsewhere in Europe during the 1930s, whose members were mostly Jews, was a personal tragedy for each of them. Nevertheless, it led to a new way of thinking about neurosis and psychosis throughout the English-speaking world, and immeasurably enriched psychiatry. It is significant that the Jungians of the day, who were mostly non-Jewish, were not scattered to the same extent by the Holocaust, which may partly account for the fact that Jungian ideas and methods were slow to spread. Those who were drawn to Jung had to go to Switzerland to find out more, and most of them who did so in the first half of the century were American.

Memory is a crucial tool in the practice of psychotherapy. The patient remembers a dream, his associations with it carry him further into his memory store, perhaps into long-forgotten places. Our most enduring memories, and those which tug at us through the years, are those linked to emotional events, change or development. I can remember so many beginnings and changes; the day I listened to the wind, the eternal wind of Shetland, whistling through the telegraph wires and I learned to whistle too. I remember the day and place where I became 'me'. 'I can do anything, I can go anywhere,' I thought. I was nine years old. I can remember going into a meadow, years later, and knowing that I had been there before by its scent. I remember climbing to the top of a rock in a remote part of Shetland, and there I saw a rock pipit a few feet away. We stayed still and looked at each other for a long time. Never had I felt so at one, not just with this tiny bird, but with the whole of nature.

'I remember' and 'Do you remember?' reverberate down the century. Those who gathered with a mixture of fear and excited anticipation before the two world wars of this century were very special groups. The gathering of a group of the First World War poets at Dymock in the summer of 1914 was remembered for long, and is kept alive today by the Friends of Dymock Poets. Thirteen years after that summer Wilfred Gibson (1994) wrote:

> Do you remember that still summer evening
> When in the cosy cream-washed living room
> Of the Old Nailshop, we all talked and laughed…? (p.91)

And Edward Thomas wrote 'Yes, I remember Adlestrop…' when he remembered that summer (Thomas 1974). In 1939 Kenneth and I altered our usual plan of travelling together in August. We got together a group of eight and camped in Galloway, and sat round a camp fire at night and told stories. We knew it would be the last holiday together for a long time, and dimly realised that things would never be the same again. Perhaps the most enduring 'remember' of all is in the last line of Binyon's poem *At the going down of the sun and in the morning…* (Binyon 1966). Down the years generation after generation has listened to those words and responded with the thunderous 'We will remember them' in a way that must bring joy in heaven to all who died in those vast conflicts.

Beginnings and endings are the trickiest phases in individual or group therapy. In the first session we meet as strangers, at the last we may, as a patient once said to me, feel that we have known each other all our lives. We perceive each other differently, the patient has brought his parents, his sibs, his friends, his wife and probably many other characters into the consulting room. Sometimes the room feels crowded with his family, at other times we are intimate and just the two of us. The therapist leaves his own family and friends to the imagination of his patient, his gift to his patient is himself, supported by the surroundings of his room. At the end of the analysis the patient has to say goodbye, and from then on his analyst is never again perceived like anyone else and the memories and the wisdom of therapy are part of him and work their magic for the rest of his life.

Writing this book has involved me in situations and dilemmas similar to those encountered in therapy. How often after a session the patient wishes he had said something else, or said what he did differently. And he may come to a session to tell you about an event, adding, 'If only I could have seen you then!' How often have I had a brilliant thought or idea in the middle of the night which won't come out the same the next day. And sometimes the muse tugs and badgers and drives one on, and the result doesn't look too bad. When I read Jung's *Memories, Dreams, Reflections* for the first time I realised that the process of writing it must have been a process of self-analysis. During the writing of this book I have made many connections which I had not previously understood, and made some interesting discoveries about myself. I write these last lines of the final chapter knowing that there are still many things I wish I had said, many topics still to be explored. I leave the work reluctantly, writing as I do just after the close of the 20th century. When I was a child the century was still fresh; everything which had occurred before the outbreak of war in 1914 belonged to a different age, it was 'Edwardian'. I see myself as a 20th century man, and I move reluctantly into the new century and a new millennium. No wonder our ancestors thought that the world would end at the conclusion of the first millennium. As the new century grows I expect to feel rather as I did when I left Louis' consulting room for the last time with the question running round my mind, 'Can I manage by myself?' But, of course, we are always alone in one sense, and in another, never alone. There are many people in my life and I could not do without them, but in the darkness of the night it is the unconscious which is my most reliable friend. Sometimes it terrifies me, but I know that it is absolutely reliable and that the better we know each other the greater will be my sanity and sense of wholeness.

References

Arnott, S., Wilkinson, E. and Aylard, P. (1993) 'A survey of psychotherapy experience among psychiatric registrars.' *Psychiatric Bulletin 1*, 695–698.

Barraclough, E. M. B., Bunch, J., Nelson, B. and Sainsbury, B. (1970) *The Proceedings of the Fifth International Conference on Suicide Prevention*, Vienna.

Bateson, G., Jackson, D.D., Hayley, J. and Weakland, J. (1956) 'Towards a theory of schizophrenia.' *Behavioral Science 1*, 251.

Binyon, L. (1966) 'For the fallen' In A. Quiller-Couch (ed) *The Oxford Book of English Verse*. Oxford: Clarendon Press.

Box, M. (ed) (1967) *The Trial of Marie Stopes*. London: Femina Books.

Bryant, A. (1953) *The Story of England, Vol 1: Makers of the Realm*. London: Collins.

Busch, A.K. and Johnson, W.C. (1950) 'LSD 25 as an Aid to Psychotherapy.' *Diseases of the Nervous System 11*, 241.

Chopra, R.N. (1933) *Indian Journal of Medicine 21*, 261.

Close, S. (1980) *Birth Report*. London NFER.

Colonna, M.T. (1980) 'Lilith and the black moon.' *Journal of Analytical Psychology 25, 4, 325–350*.

Crocket, R., Sandison, R..A. and Walk, A. (eds) (1963) *Hallucinogenic Drugs and Their Psychotherapeutic Use*. London: H.K. Lewis and Co.

Cutner, M. (1959) 'Analytic work with LSD.' *Psychiatric Quarterly 33*, 715–757.

Dell, F. and Jordan-Smith, P. (eds) (1927) *Robert Burton's* The Anatomy of Melancholy. New York: Tudor Publishing company

Dickens, C. (1892) *The Posthumous Papers of the Pickwick Club*. London: Chapman and Hall.

Eddington, A.S. (1929) *The Nature of the Physical World*. Cambridge: Cambridge University Press.

Editorial (1999) 'The physician as scientist and naturalist.' *The Lancet 354*, 9189, 30 October.

Eisner, B. (1959) *Observations on Possible Order in the Unconscious*. Read at a meeting of the Collegium Internationale for Neurology and Psychiatry (CINP), Rome.

Freud, S. (1924-1950) 'Mourning and melancholy.' In *Collected Papers IV*. London: Hogarth Press. (Originally published in 1917.)

Freud, S. (1953–1974) *The Psychopathology of Everyday Life*. In *The Standard Edition* (tr. J. Strachey), *Vol. VI*. London: Hogarth Press. (Originally published in 1901.)

Freud, S. (1953–1974) *The Standard Edition* (tr. J. Strachey) – *Vol. IV The Interpretation of Dreams I, Vol. V The Interpretation of Dreams II*, and *On Dreams*. London: Hogarth Press.

Freud, S. (Undated) *On Dreams*. Translated by M.D. Eder, with introduction by W.L. MacKenzie, London: Heinemann and Rebman.

Fromm-Reichmann, F. (1959) *Psychoanalysis and Psychotherapy: Selected Papers*. Chicago and London: University of Chicago Press.

Grimm brothers (1975) *The Robber Bridegroom*. In *The Complete Grimm Fairy Tales*. London: Routledge and Kegan Paul.

Grof, S. (1975) *Realms of the Human Unconscious*. London: Souvenir Press.

Haddock, R. (1999) 'Psychotherapy services and the NHS.' *Psychiatric Bulletin 23*, 7, 390.

Hadfield, J.A. (1923, revised 1936) *Psychology and Morals*. London: Methuen and Co.

Haggard, R. (1998) *She.* Oxford: Oxford World Classics. (Originally published in 1887.)

Hall, P. (1989) Personal communication.

Hayman, R. (1999) *A Life of Jung.* London: Bloomsbury.

Hilton, J. (1887) *Rest and Pain* (ed. W.H.A. Jacobson). Lodon: George Bell and Son.

Hoffman, E. (1997) *Lost in Translation.* London: Minerva.

Hofmann, A. (1983) *LSD, My Problem Child.* Los Angeles: Jeremy P. Tarcher, Inc.

Holmes, J. (1996) 'Psychoanalysis: An endangered species.' *Psychiatric Bulletin 20,* 6, 321.

Holmes, J. (1998) 'Allocation of scarce psychotherapeutic resources: Two landmark documents.' *Psychiatric Bulletin 22,* 2, 65.

Hunter, R. and McAlpine, I. (1963) *Three Hundred Years of Psychiatry.* Oxford: Oxford University Press.

Huxley, A. (1932) *Bare New World.* London: Chatto and Windus.

Huxley, A. (1954) *The Doors of Perception.* London: Chatto and Windus.

Hwang, K. and Drummond, L. (1996) 'Psychotherapy training and experience of successful candidates in the MRCPsych Examination.' *Psychiatric Bulletin 20,* 604–606.

Innes, M.M. (tr) (1955) *The Metamorphoses of Ovid.* Harmondsworth: Penguin Books.

Jacob, W.W. (1924) 'The monkey's paw.' In V.H. Collins (ed) *Ghosts and Marvels.* Oxford: Oxford University Press.

Jeans, J. (1929) *The Universe Around Us.* Cambridge University Press.

Jung, C.G. (1916) *The Psychology of Dreams.* Expanded 1946. In *Collected Works 8.* London: Routledge and Kegan Paul (1960).

Jung, C.G. (1954) *Collected Works 14.* London: Routledge and Kegan Paul.

Jung, C.G. (1958) *Answer to Job.* In *Collected Works 11.* London: Routledge and Kegan Paul.

Jung, C.G. (1960) *The Psychology of Dementia Praecox.* In *The Psychogenesis of Mental Disorder, Collected Works 3.* London: Routledge and Kegan Paul.

Jung, C.G. (1961) *Memories, Dreams, Reflections.* London: Collins and Routledge and Kegan Paul.

Kipling, R. (1918) *Just So Stories.* London: Macmillan.

Kipling, R. (1926) 'On the gate: A tale of 16.' In *Debits and Credits.* London: Macmillan and Co.

Klüver, H. (1928) *Mescal.* London: Kegan Paul, Trench, Trubner and Co.

Lidz, T. (1975) *The Origins and Treatment of Schizophrenic Disorders.* London: Hutchinson.

MacDonald, G. (1949) *The Princess and Curdy.* London: J.M. Dent. (Originally published in 1877)

MacDonald, G. (1949) *The Princess and the Goblin.* London: J.M. Dent. (Originally published in 1871.)

Macrae, N. (ed) (1908) *Highland Second Sight.* Dingwall: George Souter.

McDougall, J. (2000) 'Theatres of the psyche.' *The Journal of Analytical Psychology 45,* 1, 45–62.

Martin, J. (1962) 'The treatment of twelve male homosexuals with LSD.' *Acta Psychotherapeutica 10,* 394–402.

Mayer-Gross, W. (1951) 'Experimental psychoses and other mental abnormalities produced by drugs.' *British Medical Journal,* August 11, 317–321.

Mayer-Gross, W., McAdam, W. and Walker, J. (1952) 'd-Lysergic Acid Diethylamide (LSD 25) and carbohydrate metabolism: Preliminary communication.' *Nervenarzt 23,* 30.

Melechi, A. (1997) 'Acid vigil: The Michael Hollingshead Story.' In A. Melechil (ed) *Psychedelia Brittanica.* London: Turnaround.

Melechi, A. (ed) (1998) *Mindscapes.* Baildon, Yorkshire: Mono.

Michaels, R. (1975) *The Patient and the First Psychiatric Interview.* 4th Year Project, Southampton University Medical School.

Mitchell, A. (1905) *About Dreaming, Laughing and Blushing.* Edinburgh and London: William Green.

Mitchell, S.R. and Zanker, A. (1948) 'The use of music in group therapy.' *Journal of Mental Science* *94*, 737–747.

Mittwoch, A. (1987) 'Getting better, staying well.' *Group Analysis 20*, 335–342.

Morris, C. (1972) *The Discovery of the Individual, 1050–1200.* London: SPCK.

News Chronicle, 1953.

Northcote, T. (1905) *Thought Transference: A Critical and Historical Review of the Evidence for Telepathy, 1902–1903.* London: Alexander Moring.

Parry, G. and Richardson, A. (1996) *NHS Psychotherapy Services in England, Review of Strategic Policy.* London: HMSO.

Pettigrew, J. (1844) *On Superstitions Connected with the History and Practice of Medicine and Surgery.* London: Churchill.

Plath, S. (1998) *The Bell Jar.* London: Everyman's Library.

Powell, A. (1981) 'Music in the group: a musical enquiry into group-analytic psychotherapy.' *Group Analysis 14*, 3, 249.

Rees, H. (1999) 'Experiences in group-analytic psychotherapy.' *Psychiatric Bulletin 23*, 2, 101.

, M., de Shon, H.J. Hyde, R.W. and Solomon, H. (1952) 'Experimental schizophrenia-like symptoms'. *American Journal of Psychiatry 108*, 572.

Robson, B. (1987) 'A personal impression of the 14th London Workshop.' *Psychiatric Bulletin 19*, July. p.25.

Roth, A. and Fogany, P. (1996) *What Works for Whom? A Critical Review of Psychotherapy Research.* New York: Guilford Press.

Sakel, M. (1954) 'The classical Sakel shock treatment: A reappraisal.' *Journal of Clinical and Experimental Psychopathology and Quarterly Review of Psychiatry and Neurology 15*, 3,

Sandison, R. (1950) 'The psychology of electric convulsion treatment.' *Journal of Mental Science 96*, 404, 734–744.

Sandison, R. (1954) 'Psychological aspects of the LSD treatment of the neuroses.' *Journal of Mental Science 100*, 419, 508–515.

Sandison, R. (1957) 'Rauwolfia serpentina in clinical practice.' *Psychotherapy* (Calcutta) *1*, 2.

Sandison, R. (1972a) 'Depression: Illness, social disease or natural state?' *The Lancet,* June 3, 1227–1229.

Sandison, R. (1972b) 'Group training as an aid to staff development in psychiatric institutions.' *Journal of Interpersonal Development 3*, 115–139.

Sandison, R. (ed) (1979) *Report of a Symposium on Alcohol Related Problems in Shetland.* Lerwick: Shetland Health Board.

Sandison, R. (1984) *Simon's Daughter.* Lewes, Sussex: The Book Guild.

Sandison, R. (1987) 'Agents for healing in the small group.' *Group Analysis 20*, 343–349.

Sandison, R. (1991) 'The psychotic patient and psychotic conflict in group analysis.' *Group Analysis 24*, 73–83.

Sandison, R. (1993) 'The problem of good and evil.' *Group Analysis 26*, 203–212.

Sandison, R. (1994) 'Working with schizophrenics individually and in groups: Understanding the psychotic process.' *Group Analysis 27*, 391–406.

Sandison, R. (1995) 'Consciousness in the 20th century: The rôle of the group.' *Group Analysis 28*, 339–353.

Sandison, R. (1997) *Christopher Sandison of Eshaness (1781–1870): Diarist in an Age of Social Change.* Lerwick: The Shetland Times.

Sandison, R. and Chance, E. (1948) 'The Measurement of the Structure and Behaviour of Therapeutic Groups.' *Journal of Mental Science 94*, 397, 749–763.

Sandison, R., Mitchell, S., Chance, E. and Scott, R. D. (1948) 'The practice of impatient group therapy.' A collection of papers by several members of the staff of Warlingham Park Hospital, delivered at a hospital staff conference. (Not published)

Sandison, R., Spencer, A.M. and Whitelaw, J.D.A. (1954) 'The Therapeutic Value of Lysergic Acid Diethylamide in mental illness.' *Journal of Mental Science 100*, 419, 491–507.

Sandison, R., Whitelaw, E. and Currie, J.D.C. (1960) 'Clinical trials with Melleril (TP 21) in the treatment of schizophrenia.' *The Journal of Mental Science 106*, 443, 732–741.

Sandison, R. and Sevitt, M. (1977) 'The birth and early life of a psychotherapy department: Part 1.' *Group Analysis 10*, 2, 156–168. Part 2, *Group Analysis 10*, 3, 258–264.

Scott, R.D. (1950) 'The psychology of insulin coma treatment.' *British Journal of Medical Psychology 23*, 15–44.

Servadio, E. (1964) 'Drug-provoked (psychedelic) experiences as final steps in training analysis' (Rome). Unpublished.

Stoll, W.A (1947) 'Lysergsäure-diäthylamid: Ein Phasticum aus der Mutterkorngruppe.' *Schweizer Archiv fur Neurologie und Psychiatrie 60*, 1–45. Translated for the author by Dr Ruth Hofmann.

Stopes, M. (1923) *Married Love: A New Contribution to the Solution of Sex Difficulties*. London: G.P. Putnam.

Storr, A. (1999) 'Jung's search for a substitute for lost faith.' *Journal of Analytical Psychology 44*, 4, 532–537.

Summers, J. (1989) *Soho*. London: Bloomsbury.

Thomas, E. (1974) 'Adlestrop.' In *Collected Poems*. London: Faber and Faber.

Tillich, P. (1952) *The Courage to Be*. New Haven: Yale University Press.

von Franz, M.L. (1970) *An Introduction to the Psychology of Fairy Tales*. Zurich: Spring Publications.

Whitaker, H. (1964) 'Lysergic Acid Diethylamide in psychotherapy – Part 1: Clinical aspects.' *The Medical Journal of Australia*, January 4, 5-8, 37-41.

Wing, J.K. (1923) 'Social and familial factors in the causation and treatment of schizophrenia.' *Biochemical Scociety Specialist Publications I*, 153–163.

Wing, J.K. and Brown, G.W. (1970) *Institutionalisation and Schizophrenia*. Cambridge: Cambridge University Press.

Winnicott, D.W. (1971) *Playing and Reality*. London: Tavistock.

Winnicott, D.W. (1980) *The Piggle*. Harmondsworth: Penguin Books.

Wooster, G. and Boakes, J. (1989) The 16th London Workshop, 3–7 January. 'Some are more equal than others – Exploring envy and jealousy in the group.' *Psychiatric Bulletin 24*, June.

Zinkin, H., Gordon, R. and Haynes, J. (eds) (1998) *Dialogue in the Analytic Setting*. London and Philadelphia: Jessica Kingsley Publishers.

Subject Index

Author
Index